Oxford
Handbook of
Diabetes

Dose schedules are being continually revised and new side effects recognized. Oxford University Press makes no representation, express or implied, that the drug dosages in this book are correct. For theses reasons the reader is strongly urged to consult the pharmaceutical company's printed instructions before administering any of the drugs recommended in this book.

Oxford Handbook of Diabetes

Helen E Turner
and
John A H Wass

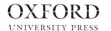

OXFORD
UNIVERSITY PRESS

Great Clarendon Street, Oxford OX2 6DP

Oxford University Press is a department of the University of Oxford.
It furthers the University's objective of excellence in research, scholarship,
and education by publishing worldwide in

Oxford New York

Auckland Bangkok Buenos Aires Cape Town Chennai Dar es Salaam Delhi
Hong Kong Istanbul Karachi Kolkata Kuala Lumpur Madrid Melbourne
Mexico City Mumbai Nairobi São Paulo Taipei Tokyo Toronto

with an associated company in Berlin

Oxford is a registered trade mark of Oxford University Press
in the UK and in certain other countries

Published in the United States
by Oxford University Press Inc., New York

© Oxford University Press, 2002

First published 2002

Merck Serono edition printed 2007

A catalogue record for this title is available from the British Library

Library of Congress Cataloging in Publication Data
Oxford handbook of endocrinology and diabetes / edited by Helen E. Turner and
John A.H. Wass.

1. Endocrinology–Handbooks, manuals, etc. 2. Diabetes–Handbooks, manuals,
etc. I. Turner, Helen, 1967– II. Wass, John.

RC649. O96 2001   616.4–dc21   2001052102

ISBN 978–0–19–923983–2

10 9 8 7 6 5 4 3 2 1

Typeset by EXPO Holdings, Malaysia
Printed in Italy
on acid-free paper by LegoPrint S.p.a

Preface

Our aim with this handbook is to provide a readily assimilable 'white coat pocket' book on diabetes, which is complementary to the *Oxford Textbook of Endocrinology and Diabetes*. Our target audience is trainees and also the trained who may have the occasional mental blank.

We are grateful to our contributors for their excellent and timely efforts and we are particularly grateful to Richard Sheaves for his considerable help in planning the book.

We have necessarily been didactic, but in order to minimize the effects of personal idiosyncrasies, we have sent each chapter to two external referees. Their names are recorded elsewhere. We are very grateful indeed to this panel of experts and for the enormous trouble that they have taken in going through the manuscript with the utmost care.

We regard this volume as the start of an evolutionary process and the first of many editions. We encourage readers to write with constructive comments and suggestions.

Helen Turner
John Wass
Department of Endocrinology
Oxford Centre for Diabetes, Endocrinology and Metabolism
Radcliffe Infirmary
Oxford
UK

March 2002

Acknowledgements

We would like to record our sincere thanks to the following friends and colleagues for their review and advice on various sections:

Professor A B Atkinson, Metabolic Unit, Royal Victoria Hospital, Belfast

Dr JS Bevan, Department of Endocrinology, Aberdeen Royal Infirmary, Aberdeen

Dr P M Bouloux, Department of Endocrinology, Royal Free Hospital, London

Dr P E Clayton, Department of Child Health, Royal Manchester Children's Hospital, Manchester

Dr G S Conway, Cobbold Laboratories, Middlesex Hospital, London

Dr N Finer, Department of Endocrinology, Luton and Dunstable Hospital, Luton

Professor J A Franklyn, Department of Medicine, Queen Elizabeth Hospital, Birmingham

Professor S Franks, Department of Endocrinology, St Mary's Hospital Medical School, London

Professor AB Grossman, Department of Endocrinology, St Bartholomew's Hospital, London

Professor R R Holman, Diabetes Trials Unit, Oxford Centre for Diabetes, Endocrinology and Metabolism, Radcliffe Infirmary, Oxford

Professor D Hosking, Division of Mineral Medicine, City Hospital, Nottingham

Dr D R Matthews, Oxford Centre for Diabetes, Endocrinology and Metabolism, Radcliffe Infirmary, Oxford

Dr A Neil, Oxford Centre for Diabetes, Endocrinology and Metabolism, Radcliffe Infirmary, Oxford

Professor CWG Redman, Nuffield Department of Obstetrics and Gynaecology, John Radcliffe Hospital, Oxford

Professor M O Savage, Department of Paediatric Endocrinology, St Bartholomew's Hospital, London

Dr B Shine, Department of Biochemistry, John Radcliffe Hospital, Oxford

Professor PM Stewart, Department of Medicine, Queen Elizabeth Hospital, Edgbaston, Birmingham

Professor R Thakker, Nuffield Department of Medicine, John Radcliffe Hospital, Oxford and Oxford Centre for Diabetes, Endocrinology and Metabolism, Radcliffe Infirmary, Oxford

Professor A P Weetman, Clinical Science Centre, Northern General Hospital, Sheffield

Professor F Wu, Department of Endocrinology, Manchester Royal Infirmary, Manchester.

Contents

Foreword

In this day and age of the internet, multimedia materials, and inter-active CDs it is easy to forget that old-fashioned method of learning and education – the book. I suspect that many like myself still prefer to look things up in a book rather than wrestle with a computer. There are two main types of book – the reference book and the handy manual. The former is useful when you wish to review a topic in depth or look up an uncommon condition or presentation, but often one wants to check a simple detail, for example a reference range or diag-nostic criterion. Handbooks are ideal for this as they can be carried around or kept easily available. The current work is an ideal example. It is packed with useful information and is very up to date – some-thing not shared by most major textbooks. It is ideally suited for the specialist registrar in endocrinology and diabetes – and even more so for the ageing consultant. It will also be useful in general practice with specific regard to the diabetes and thyroid sections. This is extremely important with the development of primary care diabetes clinics and the explosive rise in prevalence of diabetes, particularly in non-Europeans. It contains many helpful practical nuggets and will, I am sure, be required briefcase or pocket content. It fills a gap in an important area of clinical practice. The authors and publishers are to be commended – I just hope that the next edition has already been planned.

Professor Sir George Alberti
President
Royal College of Physicians
London, UK

Contributors

David B Dunger Department of Paediatrics, University of Cambridge, Cambridge, UK

Mohgah Elsheikh Department of Diabetes and Endocrinology, Royal Berkshire Hospital, Reading, Berkshire, UK

Ken Ong Department of Paediatrics, University of Cambridge, Cambridge, UK

Mahesh Sathiavageeswaran Department of Endocrinology, Oxford Centre for Diabetes, Endocrinology and Metabolism, Radcliffe Infirmary, Oxford OX2 6HE, UK

Barry M Seemungal Department of Endocrinology, Oxford Centre for Diabetes, Endocrinology and Metabolism, Radcliffe Infirmary, Oxford OX2 6HE, UK

Peter Selby Department of Medicine, Manchester Royal Infirmary, Oxford Road, Manchester M13 9WL, UK

Richard Sheaves Division of Medicine, Jersey Hospital, Jersey, Channel Islands

Kevin P Shotliff Department of Medicine, Kingston Hospital, Kingston upon Thames, Surrey KT2 7QB, UK

Garry D Tan Oxford Centre for Diabetes, Endocrinology and Metabolism, Radcliffe Infirmary, Oxford OX2 6HE, UK

Helen E Turner Department of Endocrinology, Oxford Centre for Diabetes, Endocrinology and Metabolism, Radcliffe Infirmary, Oxford OX2 6HE, UK

John A H Wass Department of Endocrinology, Oxford Centre for Diabetes, Endocrinology and Metabolism, Radcliffe Infirmary, Oxford OX2 6HE, UK

H John Wong Department of Clinical Biochemistry, Kingston Hospital, Kingston upon Thames, Surrey KT2 7QB, UK

Abbreviations

ACE	angiotensin converting enzyme
ACEI	angiotensin converting enzyme inhibitor
AD	autosomal dominant
ADA	American Diabetes Association
AGE	advanced glycation end-products
ALT	alanine transaminase
BP	blood pressure
CHD	coronary heart disease
CMV	cytomegalovirus
CSII	continuous subcutaneous insulin infusion
DCCT	Diabetes Control and Complications Trial
DI	diabetes insipidus
DIDMOAD	*d*iabetes *i*nsipidus, *DM*, *o*ptic *a*trophy + sensorineural *d*eafness (Wolfram's syndrome)
DVLA	Driver and Vehicle Licensing Agency
EE2	ethinyl oestradiol
ESR	erythrocyte sedimentation rate
ESRF	end-stage renal failure
ETDRS	Early Treatment of Diabetic Retinopathy Study
FBC	full blood count
FCHL	familial combined hyperlipidaemia
FH	familial hypercholesterolaemia
FSH	follicle stimulating hormone
GAD	glutamic acid decarboxylase
GFR	glomerular filtration rate
GH	growth hormone
GI	gastrointestinal
HDL	high-density lipoprotein
HLA	human leukocyte antigens
HNF	hepatic nuclear factor

IDDM	insulin dependent diabetes mellitus (type 1)
IFG	impaired fasting hyperglycaemia
IGF-I	insulin-like growth factor-1
IGT	impaired glucose tolerance
IRMA	intraretinal microvascular abnormalities
ITT	insulin tolerance test
IU	international units
IUGR	intrauterine growth retardation
LDL	low-density lipoprotein
LFT	liver function test
LH	luteinizing hormone
MHC	major histocompatibility complex
MI	myocardial infarct
MODY	maturity onset diabetes of the young
MRSA	methicillin-resistant *Staphylococcus aureus*
NGF	nerve growth factor
NIDDM	non-insulin dependent diabetes mellitus (type 2)
NVD	new vessels on the disc (diabetic retinopathy)
NVE	new vessels elsewhere (diabetic retinopathy)
OCP	oral contraceptive pill
OGTT	oral glucose tolerance test
PAI	platelet activator inhibitor
PPAR	peroxisome proliferator activated receptor
TG	triglycerides
TGF	transforming growth factor
UKPDS	UK Prospective Diabetes Study
VEGF	vascular endothelial growth factor
VLDL	very high-density lipoprotein
WHO	World Health Organization

Chapter 1
Diabetes: classification and diagnosis

Background

Diabetes mellitus (DM) is characterized by an elevated blood glucose. The classification of diabetes has also recently been revised to give an idea of the underlying cause or defect. Currently 2–6% of the UK population have diabetes but only 1/2 to 2/3 are thought to be diagnosed. Worldwide 100 million people have diabetes and this will probably double by the year 2010.

Current classification of diabetes

Type 1 (5–25% of cases): pancreatic islet β cell deficiency

* autoimmune – associated with anti-glutamic acid decarboxylase (GAD), islet cell, and insulin antibodies
* idiopathic

Type 2 (75–95% of cases): defective insulin action or secretion

* insulin resistance
* insulin secretory defect

Others

* Genetic defects of β cell function
– maturity onset diabetes of the young (MODY)
– chromosome 20, HNF4α (MODY 1)
– chromosome 7, glucokinase (MODY 2)
– chromosome 12, HNF1α (MODY 3)
– chromosome 13, IPF-1 (MODY 4)
  – mitochondrial DNA 3242 mutation
  – others
* Genetic defects of insulin action
  – type A insulin resistance
  – leprechaunism (type 2 diabetes, intrauterine growth retardation + dysmorphic features)
  – Rabson–Mendenhall syndrome (DM + pineal hyperplasia + acanthosis nigricans)
  – lipoatrophic diabetes
  – others
* Diseases of the exocrine pancreas
  – pancreatitis
  – trauma/surgery (pancreatectomy)
  – neoplasia
  – pancreatic destruction, e.g. cystic fibrosis, haemochromatosis
  – others (*continued on page 5*)

Diagnosis

DM is a biochemical diagnosis. In 1985 the World Health Organization (WHO) revised its guidelines to give a diagnostic template based on a 75 g oral glucose tolerance test (OGTT) which remained the gold standard until it was futher revised in 2000. The venous plasma glucose levels for this are shown on p. 7. In 1997 the American Diabetes Association (ADA) suggested lowering the normal fasting plasma glucose level to <6.0 mmol/L and the diabetic level to >7.0 mmol/L. The aim of this was to reduce the need for an OGTT and the 2 h post glucose load measurement. A fasting glucose would therefore be the diagnostic test of choice and only pregnant women would expect to have a 2 h postprandial level checked. A diagnosis of diabetes would be made in any symptomatic person with a random blood glucose >11.1 mmol/L. Asymptomatic patients or those with intercurrent illness would still require a further abnormal result before a diagnosis of diabetes could be made.

Current classification of diabetes (*continued*)

- Endocrinopathies
  - Cushing's syndrome
  - acromegaly
  - phaeochromocytoma
  - glucagonoma
  - hyperthyroidism
  - somatostatinoma
  - others
- Drug or chemical induced
- Infections
  - congenital rubella or cytomegalovirus (CMV)
  - others
- Uncommon forms of immune-mediated diabetes
  - anti-insulin receptor antibodies
  - stiff man syndrome (type 1 diabetes, rigidity of muscles, painful spasms)
  - others
- Other genetic syndromes associated with diabetes
  - Down's syndrome
  - Klinefelter's syndrome
  - Lawrence–Moon–Biedl syndrome
  - myotonic dystrophy
  - Prader–Willi syndrome
  - Turner's syndrome
  - Wolfram's syndrome (or DIDMOAD – *d*iabetes *i*nsipidus, *DM*, *o*ptic *a*trophy + sensorineural *d*eafness)
  - others
- Gestational diabetes.

Classification

The first accepted classification of diabetes was drawn up by WHO and modified in 1985. The original classification suggested just two major groups and an 'others' group. These two main groups are:

• insulin dependent DM (IDDM) or type 1
• non-insulin dependent DM (NIDDM) or type 2

In 1997, at the same time as the ADA proposed a change to the diagnostic criteria, an alteration in the classification to include both clinical stage and aetiology was also suggested. The clinical staging is from normal glucose tolerance through impaired glucose tolerance (IGT) and/or impaired fasting hyperglycaemia (IFG) and on to frank DM, which is split into non-insulin requiring, insulin requiring for control, and insulin requiring for survival. The aetiological groups are shown in the list on p. 3. The suggestion is to remove the terms IDDM and NIDDM and to expand the type 1, type 2, and 'others' groups to give a better idea of underlying cause.

Table 1.1 WHO classification

		Venous plasma glucose (mmol/L)
Normal	Fasting	<6.0
	and	
	2 h post-prandial	<7.8
Diabetes	Fasting	>7.0
	or	
	2 h post-prandial	>11.1
IGT	Fasting	<7.0
	and	
	2 h post-prandial	7.8–11.1
IFG	Fasting	6.0–6.9

Table 1.2 Spectrum of diabetic disorders in Europe

Idiopathic type 2	50%
Predominant ß cell defect (type 1 like)	18%
Type 1	15%
Latent autoimmune diabetes in adults (late onset type 1, positive GAD antibodies)	10%
MODY	5%
Mitochondrial diabetes with deafness	1%
Insulin receptor defects	<1%

Adapted from Groop (1998).

Table 1.3 Differences between type 1 and type 2 diabetes

	Type 1 diabetes	Type 2 diabetes
Peak age of onset	12 years	60 years
UK prevalence	0.25%	5–7% (10% of those >65 years of age)
Aetiology	Autoimmune	Combination of insulin resistance, ß cell destruction and ß cell dysfunction
Initial presentation	Polyuria, polydypsia, and weight loss with ketoacidosis	Hyperglycaemic symptoms but often with complication of diabetes
Treatment	Diet and insulin from outset	Diet with or without oral hypoglycaemic agents or insulin

Genetics

Type 1 patients

The overall lifetime risk in a white population of developing type 1 diabetes is only 0.4%, but this rises to:

* 1–2% if your mother has it
* 3–6% if your father has it
* siblings have about a 6% risk
* monozygotic twins have a 36% concordance rate.

Islet cell antibodies are seen in 3% of Oxford schoolchildren but in 40% of monozygotic twins and 6% of siblings of type 1 patients. A genetic predisposition is therefore suggested, but this also highlights the importance of environmental triggers as not all those with antibodies go on to get diabetes. Genetic predisposition accounts for 1/3 of susceptibility to type 1 diabetes.

Although several different regions of the human genome are linked to the development of type 1 diabetes, the most common are the major histocompatibility complex (MHC) antigens/human leukocyte antigens (HLA). Over 90% of type 1 patients in this country have either HLA-DR3, DR4, or both. Certain variants of the DQβ1 or DQA1 gene result in the expression of susceptible alleles of DR3/DR4. Interestingly this association is not true in all races, notably the Japanese.

There are currently 10 distinct genetic areas (IDDM1–IDDM10) known to be linked to type 1 diabetes; some relate to MHC genes, others to the insulin gene region. MHC antigens commonly found in those with type 1 diabetes, and felt to predispose to it, are B15, B8, and DQ8. The DR2, DQ6, and DQ18 genes appear to be protective. Linkage studies have suggested type 1 susceptibility genes on chromosomes:

* 6q (also known as IDDM5)
* 11p (IDDM2)
* 11q (IDDM4)
* 15q (IDDM3).

These genetic variations may help to explain susceptibility, but their link to the increased levels of islet cell antibodies, anti-glutamic acid decarboxylase (GAD) antibodies, and anti-tyrosine phosphatase antibodies (anti-IA-2 antibodies) often seen soon after diagnosis is less clearly decided. These three antibodies, if all are present, give a non-diabetic individual an 88% chance of developing type 1 diabetes in the next 10 years.

Maturity onset diabetes of the young
MODY 1 (HNF4α)

* Accounts for <0.0001% of all type 2 patients and about 5% of cases of MODY.
* Usually presents in adolescence or early adulthood <25 years of age
* Can give severe hyperglycaemia with 20% needing insulin therapy and 40% oral agents
* Results in a high frequency of microvascular complications.
* Inherited as an autosomal dominant with a defect on chromosome 20q resulting in altered activity of the hepatic nuclear factor (HNF)4α gene which is a positive regulator of HNF1α. This is a transcription factor found in the liver and β cells of the pancreas where it acts as a transactivater of the insulin gene in rat models.

MODY 2 (glucokinase)

* Accounts for <0.2% of type 2 patients and 10% of cases of MODY.
* Presents in early childhood
* Gives only mild hyperglycaemia and therefore infrequent microvascular complications with 90% controlled on diet alone and insulin usually only needed when they become pregnant.
* Autosomally dominantly inherited with a defect in the glucokinase gene on chromosome 7 resulting in altered glucose sensing in the β cells of the pancreas and impaired hepatic production of glycogen.

MODY 3 (HNF1α)

* Affects 1–2% of type 2 patients and accounts for 70% of MODY patients.
* Presents in adolescence or early adulthood (peaks around 21 years of age).
* Causes severe hyperglycaemia and frequent microvascular complications; 1/3 require insulin therapy and 1/3 require oral agents.
* Linked to a mutation on chromosome 12q24 which directly alters HNF1α activity. How this causes type 2 diabetes is not fully understood.

Type 2 patients

In type 2 patients the concordance between monozygotic twins for diabetes is much higher (60–100%, versus 36% for type 1) but the rate amongst dizygotic twins is much less, suggesting a much stronger genetic element in its aetiology than for type 1 diabetes. Unlike type 1 patients, however, those with type 2 do not seem to have the same HLA-linked genes. In most families this appears to be polygenic, although the much less common maturity onset diabetes of the young (MODY) is autosomal dominant but only accounts for a few percent of all type 2 patients. MODY is currently split into four types, with type 4 accounting for 15% of cases and currently accounting for those that do not fit into types 1–3, although a chromosome 13 defect in the insulin promoter factor 1 gene may fall into this group.

Other recognized genetic subtypes of type 2 diabetes include *mitochondrial diabetes*, which effects 1–3% of type 2 patients and is maternally transmitted. It is associated with deafness and other neurological abnormalities. *Insulin resistance* is an important part of type 2 diabetes and rare genetic defects causing this are recognized. A 40% reduction in the biological effect of any given insulin molecule is suggested by clamp studies in type 2 patients, but these rarer genetic syndromes may result in a more severe picture.

References and further reading

Alberti KGMM, Zimmet PZ, for the WHO consultation. Definition, diagnosis and classification of DM and its complications. Part 1: Diagnosis and classification of DM. Provisional report of a WHO consultation. *Diabetic Medicine* 1998; 15: 539–553.

Alcolado JC, Thomas AW. Maternally inherited DM: the role of mitochondrial DNA defects. *Diabetic Medicine* 1995; 12(2):102–108.

Groop LC. Prediction and prevention of type 2 DM. *Topical Endocrinology* 1998;10: 13–16.

Hattersley AT. Maturity onset diabetes of the young (MODY). *Baillière's Clinical Paediatrics* 1996; 4(4): 663–680.

Robinson S, Kessling A. Diabetes secondary to genetic disorders. *Baillière's Clinical Endocrinology and Metabolism* 1992; 6: 867–898.

Chapter 2

General management and treatment

Background

After diagnosis all patients with diabetes need to see a dietitian and a diabetes nurse specialist and have a full medical assessment. The first priority is dietary advice, which should always take into account the patient's circumstances and culture and be individually tailored in order to be achievable.

Assessment of the newly diagnosed patient

History
- duration of symptoms, e.g. thirst, polyuria, weight loss
- possible secondary causes of diabetes, e.g. acromegaly
- family history
- presence of complication of diabetes
- risk factors for developing complications e.g. smoking, hypertension, hyperlipidaemia.

Examination
- body mass index (BMI)
- clues for secondary causes
- cardiovascular system (especially BP + peripheral pulses)
- signs of autonomic and peripheral neuropathy
- eyes – for retinopathy

Investigations
Initial investigations will be modified by the history and examination but as a minimum should include:
- blood tests for urea and electrolytes, liver and thyroid function, and a full lipid profile
- urine tests for ketones, macro- and (if negative) microalbuminuria
- an ECG in all type 2 patients.

Treatment
In type 1 patients, insulin therapy is mandatory along with dietary advice and standard diabetes education. The education of all newly diagnosed patients is intended to provide an incentive for good compliance. A full education package should include:
- an explanation as to what diabetes is and what it means to the patient
- aims of treatment, e.g. rationale of reducing complications and exact values to aim for

- types of treatment – not just drugs but also dietary advice and lifestyle modification such as increased physical activity, stopping smoking, and reducing alcohol intake
- self monitoring, e.g. both the method(s) of doing this, the reasons for doing it, and what to do with the results
- an idea of some chronic complications of diabetes and what to look out for, e.g. a chiropodist's input and review is advised, especially for type 2 patients
- advice regarding DVLA, insurance companies, and Diabetes U.K.

All type 2 patients should be considered for such an educational package. In most the next step is to try diet, exercise, and weight reduction (if obese, which most will be) before initiating drug therapy if control is not adequate. If this fails to improve control adequately after 3 months, consider oral therapy with *metformin* in the overweight and *sulfonylureas* in the lean.

After the initial assessment all patients should be put into a formal review system, whether by their GP or in a hospital diabetic clinic, for further education, maintenance of good control, and complication screening.

Dietary advice

In the overweight patient (e.g. BMI >25) a reduction in total intake to aid weight reduction is also required. A standard diabetic diet should aim to have

- <10% of its energy in the form of saturated fat (<8% if hyper-lipidaemic)
- <30% from all fats
- 50–60% as carbohydrate which is mostly complex high fibre
- sugar limited to about 25 g/day
- sodium content <6 g/day in most people or <3 g/day if hypertensive.

Alcohol is a significant source of calories, and a reduction in the overweight or hypertriglyceridaemic patient is advisable.

Oral hypoglycaemic agents

Sulfonylureas

These agents are used as first line treatment in non-obese patients with type 2 diabetes.

- The first generation agents *chlorpropamide*, *tolbutamide*, and *tolazamide* are still used today.
- Second generation agents such as *glibenclamide*, *gliclazide*, and *glipizide* are now more commonly used.
- Third generation agents such as *glimepiride* have recently become available.

Mode of action

Sulfonylureas act by stimulating a receptor on the surface of β cells, closing a potassium channel and opening a calcium channel with subsequent insulin release. A doubling of glucose-stimulated insulin secretion can be expected with both first and second phase insulin secretion affected. This results in a 1–2% reduction in HbA1c long term.

Side-effects

These are hypoglycaemia and weight gain. In the UK Prospective Diabetes Study (UKPDS) the mean weight gain seen after 10 years of therapy was 2.3 kg while the incidence of major hypoglycaemic events was 0.4–0.6%/year. Occasional skin reactions, alterations in liver function tests, and minor gastrointestinal symptoms may be more important. Also avoid sulfonylureas in porphyria.

Biguanides

Metformin is first line therapy in the obese type 2 diabetic and is also used in some insulin-treated, insulin-resistant, overweight subjects to reduce insulin requirements. The UKPDS showed significantly better results from metformin for complications and mortality compared to other therapies in the overweight type 2 diabetic. Although a 1–2 kg weight loss is seen initially, UKPDS data suggests it does not significantly alter weight over a 10 year period.

Mode of action

Metformin works by decreasing hepatic gluconeogenesis and increasing muscle glucose uptake/metabolism, so increasing insulin sensitivity. With long term use a 0.8–2.0% reduction in HbA1c can be expected.

Table 2.1 Properties of sulfonylureas

Sulfonylurea	Length of action	Begins working within	Daily dose (mg)
Glibenclamide	16–24 h	2–4 h	2.5–15
Glicazide	10–24 h	2–4 h	40–320
Gliclazide MR	10–24 h	2–4 h	30–120
Glipizide	6–24 h	2–4 h	2.5–20
Chlorpropamide	24–72 h	2–4 h	100–500
Tolbutamide	6–10 h	2–4 h	500–2000
Glimepiride		2–4 h	1–6

Table 2.2 Biguanides and prandial glucose regulators

Drug	Length of action	Begins working within	Daily dose (mg)
Metformin	24–36 h	2.5 h	500–2000
Repaglinide	4–6 h	<1 h	0.5–16
Nateglinide	–	–	180–540

Side-effects/contraindications

Contraindicated in patients with renal (creatinine >140 nmol/L), hepatic, or cardiac impairment, or who consume significant alcohol. Gastrointestinal side-effects include nausea, epigastric discomfort, and diarrhoea and occur in up to 1/2 of patients in the first 1–2 weeks of treatment, but are usually transient. If the starting dose is low (e.g. 500 mg once daily) most people develop a tolerance to these and are able to take higher doses; <5% are totally intolerant. Rarely skin rashes and lactic acidosis occur. The latter, when seen, is usually in patients with hepatic, renal, or cardiac impairment. Using radiological contrast media with metformin is associated with an increased risk of lactic acidosis and therapy should be stopped for a few days before such investigations. Lactic acidosis occurs very infrequently e.g. 0.024–0.15 cases/1000 patient years in a Swedish study. *Phenformin* was used in the past but was withdrawn due to an increased risk of lactic acidosis. Although it is known to reduce folic acid and vitamin B_{12} absorption this is not usually a problem clinically with metformin.

Prandial glucose regulators

This new form of therapy can be used in type 2 patients who have inadequate control on diet or metformin. *Repaglinide* is a non-sulfonylurea oral hypoglycaemic agent which stimulates the secretion of insulin from pancreatic β cells. It works on separate parts of the β cell sulfonylurea receptor from the sulfonylureas. Its use results in an approximate 0.6–2% reduction in HbA1c levels. Its very short duration of action reduces the risk of hypoglycaemia compared to some sulfonylureas. It should not, however, be used in patients with renal or hepatic impairment and may result in hepatic dysfunction so periodic liver function test monitoring is required.

α-Glucosidase inhibitors

Used in type 2 patients who have inadequate control on diet or other oral agent alone. When taken with food acarbose reduces post prandial glucose peaks by inhibiting the digestive enzyme α-glucosidase which normally breaks carbohydrates into their monosaccharide components, thus retarding glucose uptake from the intestine and reducing postprandial glucose peaks. Some improvement in lipids has also been reported.

These undigested carbohydrates then pass into the large intestine where bacteria metabolize them, which may explain the common side-effects of postprandial fullness/bloating, abdominal pain, flatulence, and diarrhoea. Starting at 50 mg once daily and gradually increasing the dose at 2–3 weekly intervals improves tolerance to this therapy. Less commonly, jaundice and elevated hepatic transaminase levels can also be seen. In the UK PDS adding *acarbose* to other therapies resulted in a further 0.5% drop in HbA1c.

Table 2.3 Oral hypogylcaemic agents: summary

Class	Mechanism of action	Expected reduction in HbA1c (%)
Sulfonylureas	Stimulate pancreatic insulin secretion	1.5–2.5
Biguanides	Increases muscle glucose uptake and metabolism; decreases hepatic gluconeogenesis	0.8–2.0
Prandial glucose regulators	Stimulate pancreatic insulin secretion	0.5–1.9
α-Glucosidase inhibitors	Inhibits a digestive enzyme	0.4–0.7
Thiazolidinediones	Activate PPAR-γ receptor	0.6–1.5

Thiazolidinediones

This novel class of drugs act as insulin sensitizing agents by activating the peroxisome proliferator activated receptor (PPAR-γ) which stimulates gene transcription for glucose transporter molecules such as Glut 1. The first of this class was *troglitazone* which reduces insulin requirements by up to 30% and HbA1c by 1% either when used alone or in combination with other oral agents. This was withdrawn soon after its UK launch because of reports of hepatotoxicity but is still being used in other countries. Other agents such as *rosiglitazone* and *pioglitazone*, are now available in the UK. Their main side-effect is hepatotoxicity, and normal liver function before starting therapy with monthly liver function test (LFT) for the first year seems sensible.

Indications

Type 2 diabetes, oral combination with metformia or a sulfonylurea

Dose

- Rosiglitazone 4–8 mg/day
- Pioglitazone 15–30 mg/day

Side-effects

- Fluid retention
- Hepertotoxicity

Insulin

Insulin is required in all patients with type 1 diabetes, and some with type 2, for the preservation of life; in other type 2 patients it is needed to achieve better glycaemic/metabolic control or for the relief of hyperglycaemic symptoms. Most insulin is in a biosynthetic human form (from yeast or bacteria) at a standard concentration: U100 (100 units/mL). Some countries still supply U40 and U80 strengths, so care should be taken with patients from abroad. There is also a sizable minority of patients taking bovine or porcine insulins. Bovine insulin is extracted from cattle pancreas and is more antigenic than both human and porcine alternatives and so gives more lipohypertrophy and lipoatrophy.

Insulin can currently only be given by i/v or s/c routes, although inhaled formulations may soon be available. Standard insulins come as 10 mL vials for use with a 0.5 mL or 1.0 mL syringe or as 1.5 mL or 3.0 mL cartridges for use in pen devices. The insulin itself is un-modified/neutral or mixed with agents such as zinc to alter its onset of action, peak effect, and duration of action. Thre are >30 types of insulin preparation available, which should allow full 24 h cover for a wide variety of lifestyles.

The main problems with all insulin regimens are weight gain and hypoglycaemia. The later occurring overnight can be troublesome, especially as the patient may not know it has occurred and because of the counter-regulatory hormone response (the *Somogyi phenomenon*) just reacts to the hyperglycaemia the next morning by increasing their evening insulin. Occasional 3 a.m. blood glucose levels may help sort this out. Care with alcohol and adjustments of insulin and pre-bed snacks if nocturnal physical activity such as sex is on the cards will also reduce nocturnal hypos.

Types of insulin

Short acting (soluble/neutral) insulins

Unmodified or neutral insulins are short acting but are not identical. Human *actrapid* has an onset 30 min after injection with a peak onset at 2–4 h and a duration of up to 6–8 h; human *velosulin* has a similar onset and duration but an earlier peak effect. All the soluble formula-tions require a 20–30 min interval between injecting and eating to be effective.

Table 2.4 Suggested aims of treatment

Fasting blood glucose	<7 mmol/L
HbA1c	<7.2% (or <6.5% in those with significant complications)
Blood pressure	<140/80 mmHg
Body mass index	20–25 ideally
Home monitoring	Capillary blood glucose estimations fasting, pre-meal, 2 h postprandially and pre bed. These will need to be frequent enough to allow alterations in treatment and assessment of adequate control. Often adequate with 3x week in stable type 2 patients and daily in stable type 1 patients.

Table 2.5 Insulin: summary

Type of insulin	Examples	Peak activity (h)	Duration of action (h)
Insulin analogue	Humalog (insulin lispro)	0.5–1.5	<6
	Insulin Aspart (NovoRapid)		
Short acting	Human Actrapid	1–3	<8
	Humulin S		
Intermediate acting	Human Insulatard		
	Humulin I		
	Human Monotard		
	Humulin Zn	4–8	<24
Long acting	Human Ultratard	6–24	<36

Insulin analogues

Insulin *lispro* (Humalog) and Insulin *Aspart* (NovoRapid) have been modified to allow injecting and eating to occur simultaneously as they have a more rapid onset of action and earlier peak effect with peak blood insulin level approximately 1.5–2.5 times that from the same dose of standard neutral human insulin. The duration of action is also shorter at 5 h and this may cause problems if there are long gaps between meals.

A long-acting analogue (Insulin Glargine) is available in parts of Europe and the USA and will soon be available in the U.K.

Intermediate acting (isophane) insulins

Insulin action can be extended by addition of protamine or zinc to give an isophane insulin with an onset of action 1–2 h after injection, a peak at 4–6 h, and a duration of action of 8–14 h. Different preparations have slightly different profiles when looking at peak effect and maximal insulin concentrations as with soluble preparations.

Long acting insulins

Insulin to which only zinc is added such as human ultratard or Humulin Zn can have an even later onset of action of 4 h, peak at 6–18 h, and last up to 24–36 h.

Biphasic/mixed insulins

Combinations of soluble/neutral and isophane insulins are now extremely popular. The amount of soluble insulin present varies from 10 to 50%, 30% being the most popular. Depending on its mono-components onset is normally at 30 min, peak effect 2–6 h, and duration 8–12 h. Insulin analogue biphasic preparations are also available with an onset, peak, and duration all slightly shorter than these.

Insulin regimes

Twice daily free mixing

Historically very popular with 2/3 isophane, 1/3 soluble, and 2/3 of both pre-breakfast and 1/3 pre-evening meal. The main problems are mixing them, and pre lunch hypos or hyperglycaemia. If on the same doses twice daily look out for pre-evening meal hyperglycaemia and increase the morning isophane dose to compensate for this, with a reduction in the morning soluble often needed to reduce pre-lunch hypoglycaemia.

Twice daily fixed mixture

Most commonly a 30% soluble/70% isophane mixture but, although this is not ideal for pre-lunch control or alterations in diet and exercise that are not preplanned, it is indicated in type 2 patients with poor control, those with significant osmotic symptoms and those in whom there is no room to increase oral agents. A suitable starting regimen is a 30/70 mixture with 2/3 pre-breakfast and 1/3 pre-evening meal. The exact doses tend to vary widely depending on insulin sensitivity but a reasonable starting regimen may be 10–15 units pre-breakfast and 5–10 units pre-evening meal.

Basal bolus regime

Soluble insulin or an insulin analogue given 3x day pre-meal with a pre-bed isophane; potentially has more flexibility with meal times, portions, and exercise than the previous regimens. The larger number of injections and the more frequent capillary blood glucose measurements needed makes it less popular with some patients.

If starting as the first type of insulin give three equal pre-meal doses and alter as required, e.g. 4–6 units is a reasonable starting dose, with 6–8 units of isophane pre-bed. If converting from a 2× day regimen reduce the total daily insulin dose by up to 10% and give 30–50% of the remainder as the bedtime isophane and split the rest evenly between the meals. Once the patient is on this regimen the evening isophane often needs to be increased to maintain adequate fasting sugars.

In patients on insulin analogues, and less often those on standard soluble insulins, a 2x daily isophane is occasionally needed especially if there is a long gap between lunch and the evening meal.

Continuous s/c insulin infusion (CSII)

Used in the USA but not commonly in the UK because of potential problems with pump failure, ketoacidosis, and cannula site infections. Soluble insulin is given continuously via a s/c cannula into the anterior abdomen.

Insulin and oral agent mixtures

In type 2 patients several combinations are occasionally used. The two most popular are bedtime insulin + daytime tablets, or more frequent insulin + metformin. In the first, oral agents continue during the day with a pre-bed isophane used to give acceptable fasting sugars pre-breakfast. Although often starting at 10 units/night, doses 5–6 times that are not infrequently needed. This regimen is complicated but is suitable if someone else such as a district nurse or relative gives the insulin. The second regimen adds up to 2 g/day of metformin to any standard insulin regimen to reduce insulin requirements and improve control without the problem of further weight gain often seen if the insulin is continually increased.

Further reading

Alberti KGMM, Gries FA *et al.* A desktop guide for the management of non-insulin dependent diabetes mellitus (NIDDM): an update. *Diabetic Medicine* 1994; 11: 899–909.

ADA position statement. Nutrition recommendations and principles for people with diabetes mellitus. *Diabetes Care* 1994; 17: 519–522.

Bailey CJ, Turner RC. Metformin. *New England Journal of Medicine* 1996; 334: 574–579.

Campbell IW. Efficacy and limitations of sulfonyureas and metformin. In: Bailey CJ, Flatt PR, eds. *New antidiabetic drugs.* Nishimura, Japan: Smith-Gordon, 1990: 33–51.

Diabetes and Nutrition Study Group of the European Association for the Study of Diabetes. Recommendations for the nutritional management of patients with diabetes mellitus. *Diabetes Nutrition and Metabolism* 1995; 8(3): 186–189.

Ratner RE. Rational insulin management of insulin-dependent diabetes. In Leslie RDG, Robbins DE, eds. *Diabetes: clinical science in practice.* Cambridge: Cambridge University Press, 1995:434–49.

UK Prospective Diabetes Study (UKPDS) Group. Intensive blood-glucose control with sulfonylureas or insulin compared with conventional treatment and risk of complications in patients with type 2 diabetes (UKPDS 33) *Lancet* 1998; 352: 837–853.

UK Prospective Diabetes Study (UKPDS) Group. Effect of intensive blood-glucose control with metformin on complications in overweight patients with type 2 diabetes (UKPDS 34) *Lancet* 1998; 352: 854–865.

Chapter 3
Diabetic eye disease

Epidemiology

Diabetic retinopathy remains the commonest cause of blindness in the working population of developed countries. Currently 2% of the UK diabetic population are thought to be registered blind, giving a person with diabetes a 10–20-fold increased risk of blindness. It is suggested that 84 000 of the 7.8 million diabetic North Americans will develop proliferative retinopathy each year and another 95 000 macular oedema.

The prevalence of diabetic retinopathy depends on the duration of diabetes, glycaemic control, blood pressure control and the racial mix of the group being examined, but about a 30% prevalence for a general diabetic population is often quoted.

In type 1 patients <2% have any lesions of diabetic retinopathy at diagnosis and only 8% have any features of it by 5 years (2% proliferative), but 87–98% have abnormalities 30 years later, 30% of these having had proliferative retinopathy. In type 2 patients 20–37% can be expected to have retinopathy at diagnosis and 15 years later 85% of those on insulin and 60% of those not taking will have abnormalities.

The 4 year incidence for proliferative retinopathy in a large North American epidemiological study was 10.5% in type 1 patients, 7.4% in older onset/type 2 patients taking insulin, and 2.3% in those not on insulin. In the UK currently maculopathy is a more common and therefore more significant sight-threatening complication of diabetes. It is suggested that 75% of those with maculopathy have type 2 diabetes and that there is a 4 year incidence of 10.4% in this group. Although type 2 patients are 10 times more likely to have maculopathy than type 1 patients, 14% of type 1 patients who become blind do so because of maculopathy.

Diabetic retinopathy, like many microvascular complications, is more common in the ethnic minorities than in Caucasians. It should also be remembered that cataracts are more common in people with diabetes and are actually the most common eye abnormality seen. These occur in up to 60% of 30–54 year olds. Other abnormalities to look for include vitreous changes such as asteroid hyalosis which occur in about 2% of patients. These are are small spheres or star-shaped opacities seen in the vitreous which appear to sparkle when illuminated under an examining light and do not normally affect vision.

Classification and features of diabetic retinopathy

- background retinopathy
  - microaneurysms
  - haemorrhages
  - hard exudates
- preproliferative retinopathy
  - soft exudates/cotton wool spots
  - intra-retinal abnormalities (IRMAs)
  - venous abnormalities (e.g. venous beading, looping, and reduplication)
- proliferative retinopathy
  - new vessels on the disc or within 1 disc diameter of it (NVD)
  - new vessels elsewhere (NVE)
  - rubeosis iridis (± neovascular glaucoma)
- maculopathy
  - haemorrhages and hard exudates in the macula area
  - reduced visual acuity with no abnormality seen

Clinical features and histological features

The classification of diabetic retinopathy is based on ophthalmoscopic examination but several other changes not seen macroscopically may explain some of these clinical findings.

One of the first histological changes seen is thickening of the capillary basement membrane and loss of the pericytes embedded in it. Both have been linked to hyperglycaemia in experimental models, with sorbitol accumulation and advanced glycation both having a role. In normal retinal capillaries there is a 1 : 1 relationship between endothelial cells and pericytes. Pericytes may control endothelial cell proliferation, maintain the structural integrity of capillaries, and regulate blood flow. Altering these roles, along with the increased blood viscosity, abnormal fibrinolytic activity, and reduced red cell deformity also seen in diabetes may lead to capillary occlusion, tissue hypoxia, and the stimulus for new vessel formation. Exactly how locally produced growth factors, altered protein kinase C, alterations in oxidative stress responses, and alterations in the autoregulation of retinal blood flow combine to cause this remains unclear but is avidly debated.

The natural progression is from background to preproliferative/premaculopathy then to proliferative retinopathy/maculopathy, and ultimately sight-threatening disease.

Background retinopathy

Capillary microaneurysms are the earliest feature seen clinically, as red 'dots'. Small intraretinal haemorrhages or 'blots' also occur, as can haemorrhage into the nerve fibre layer which are often more flame shaped. With increased capillary leakage hard exudates, which are lipid deposits, can also be seen.

Preproliferative retinopathy

A *cotton wool spot* is an infarct in the nerve fibre layer which alters axoplasmic transport in ganglion cell neurones giving an oedematous infarct seen as a pale/grey fuzzy edged lesion, which gives it its name. Intraretinal microvascular abnormalities (IRMAs) are tortuous dilated hypercellular capillaries in the retina which occur in response to retinal ischaemia. A further change seen is alternating dilatation and constriction of veins (venous beading) and other venous alterations such as duplication and loop formation. Overall there are large areas of capillary non-perfusion occurring in the absence of new vessels.

The Early Treatment of Diabetic Retinopathy Study (ETDRS) suggested that certain of these features matter and suggested a '4–2–1' rule:

- 4 quadrants of severe haemorrhages or microaneurysms
- 2 quadrants of IRMAs
- 1 quadrant with venous beading.

If you have one of these features there is a 15% risk of developing sight-threatening retinopathy within the next year; if two are present the risk rises to 45%.

Proliferative retinopathy

New vessels are formed from the retina and can grow along, into, or out from it. A scaffolding for fibrosis then forms. There are two forms of new vessels: those on the disc or within one disc diameter of the disc (NVD) and new vessels elsewhere (NVE). Both give no symptoms but cause the problems of advanced retinopathy such as haemorrhage, scar tissue formation, traction on the retina, and retinal detachment which actually results in loss of vision. That is why panretinal photo-coagulation, which can result in the regression of these new vessels, is used when they are seen.

Diabetic maculopathy

Oedema in the macula area can distort central vision and reduce visual acuity. Any of the above changes can co-exist with maculopathy. The changes seen can be:

- oedematous (clinically it may just be difficult to focus on the macula with a hand-held ophthalmoscope)
- exudative (with haemorrhages, hard exudates, and circinate exudates)
- ischaemic (capillary loss occurs but clinically the macula may look normal on direct ophthalmoscopy but unperfused area will show up on fluorescein angiography)
- any combination of these.

A ring or circinate pattern of lipid deposits suggest a focal defect which may be treated with focal laser therapy, whereas a more diffuse problem may require more extensive treatment with a macula grid of laser.

Eye screening

As so many patients can expect to develop eye complications, some of these are sight threatening, and treatment can reduce this, a suitable screening programme is advisable. Patients with diabetes should undergo ophthalmic examination eyes at least once a year. A full examination should include the following.

Visual acuity

Use a standard Snellen chart for distance and check each eye separately. Let the patient wear their glasses for the test and if vision is worse than 6/9 also check with a pinhole as this will correct for any refractive (glasses) error. If it does not correct to 6/9 or better consider more careful review; some maculopathy changes cannot be seen easily with a hand-held ophthalmoscope and an ophthalmology review may be needed. Cataracts are a more likely cause, so look carefully at the red reflex. If vision gets worse with a pinhole, assume maculopathy is there until proven otherwise.

High blood glucose readings can give myopia (difficulty in distance vision) and low blood glucose hypermetropia (difficulty in reading), although this is not universal.

Eye examination

- Dilate the pupil before looking into the eye.
  - Use *tropicamide* 1% in most cases as it dilates the pupil adequately in 15–20 min and lasts only 2–3 h.
  - In those with a dark iris you may also need *phenylephrine* (2.5%) added soon after the tropicamide to give adequate views.
  - The main reasons not to dilate are closed angle glaucoma and recent eye surgery but, as such patients are usually under an eye clinic already, most people are suitable for dilatation.
  - 1% *pilocarpine* drops can be used (although not routinely) if acuity is >6/12 after dilatation. They may speed up reversal and allow driving sooner.
- Once the pupil is dilated, look at the red reflex to check for lens opacities. Examine the anterior chamber, as although rare, rubeosis iridis is important to pick up. The vitreous is examined before examining the retina. When examining the retina use the optic disc as a landmark, follow all four arcades of vessels out from it, examine the periphery, and at the end examine the macula as this can be uncomfortably bright through a dilated pupil and if done at the

start makes it difficult for anyone to keep their eye still enough to complete the examination adequately.

Retinal photographs

It is said that although consultant diabetologists are more accurate than GPs, they still miss some cases of retinopathy when compared to the gold standard of an ophthalmologist. One way to reduce the 'false negative' rate for a screening programme is to use retinal photography as well as ophthalmoscopy. Over 90% of people can have good quality photos performed. This is usually done with 35 mm slide film although digital images are now of sufficiently good quality, require a less intense flash, and avoid the delay of having to develop film. The photographs/images obtained should then be graded/assessed by a trained observer.

When to refer

The physician performing eye screening will need good links with an interested ophthalmologist. Referral will depend on local preferences, but consider the timing and need for referral discussed in the table below.

Reasons for and timing of referral to ophthalmologist

- immediate referral
  - proliferative retinopathy, as untreated NVD carries a 40% risk of blindness in <2 years and laser treatment reduces this
  - rubeosis iridis/neovascular glaucoma
  - vitreous haemorrhage
  - advanced retinopathy with fibrous tissue or retinal detachments
- early referral (<6 weeks)
  - preproliferative changes
  - maculopathy, both for non-proliferative retinopathy involving the macula or for any haemorrhages/hard exudates within 1 disc diameter of the fovea
  - fall of >2 lines on a Snellen chart (whatever fundoscopy shows)
- routine referral
  - cataracts
  - non-proliferative retinopathy with large circinate exudates not threatening the macula/fovea

Treatment

Glycaemic control

There is good epidemiological evidence for an association between poor glycaemic control and worsening of retinopathy. The Diabetes Control and Complications Trial (DCCT) looked at intensive glycaemic control in type 1 patients over 6.5 years and showed a 76% reduction in the risk of initially developing retinopathy in the tight glycaemic group compared to the control group. The rate of progression of existing retinopathy was slowed by 54% and the risk of developing severe non-proliferative or proliferative retinopathy was reduced by 47%. The UKPDS looked at type 2 patients over a 9 year period and showed a 21% reduction in progression of retinopathy and a 29% reduction in the need for laser therapy. The long term benefits of improved glycaemic control are therefore clear.

However, the DCCT, the UKPDS, and several previous studies also showed an initial worsening of retinopathy in the first 2 years in the tight/improved glycaemic control groups, and all patients therefore need careful monitoring over this period. The long term benefits outweigh this initial risk.

Blood pressure control/therapy

There is good evidence for an association between both systolic and diastolic hypertension and retinopathy in type 1 patients, but the link may only be with systolic hypertension in type 2 patients. The UKPDS looked at blood pressure control in type 2 patients and showed that the treatment group, with a mean BP of 144/82 mmHg, when compared to the control group which had a mean of 154/87 mmHg, had a 35% reduction in the need for laser therapy. Adequate BP control, e.g. <140/80 in type 2 patients, is therefore advocated.

Using antiotensin converting enzyme inhibitors (ACEIs) as first line therapy is also suggested. Experimental evidence suggests these agents may have antiangiogenic effects by altering local growth factor levels as well as any benefit from reducing blood pressure. Studies using *enalapril* and *lisinopril* have both shown a reduction in the progression of retinopathy in type 1 patients.

Lipid control/therapy

Experimental evidence suggests oxidized low-density lipoprotein (LDL)-cholesterol may be cytotoxic for endothelial cells. Epidemiological data also suggests an association between higher LDL-cholesterol and worse diabetic retinopathy, especially maculopathy with exudates. A total cholesterol >7.0 mmol/L gives a fourfold greater risk of proliferative retinopathy than a total cholesterol <5.3 mmol/L. A worse outcome from laser therapy in those treated for maculopathy has also been seen if hyperlipidaemia is present. Aggressive lipid lowering is therefore advocated, especially in maculopathy.

Antiplatelet therapy

In view of the altered rheological properties of diabetic patients these agents have been tried, but the results are variable. No evidence that they make things worse has been shown, and some studies suggest *aspirin* and *ticlopidine* may slow the progression of retinopathy although the benefit was small.

Lifestyle advice

Although stopping smoking reduces macrovascular risk its effect on retinopathy is less clear. Alcohol consumption and physical activity also show no consistent effect.

Risk factors for developing/worsening of diabetic retinopathy

- duration of diabetes
- type of diabetes (proliferative disease is more common in type 1 and maculopathy in type 2)
- poor diabetic control
- hypertension
- diabetic nephropathy
- recent cataract surgery
- pregnancy
- alcohol (variable results which may be related to the type of alcohol involved, e.g. worse in Scotland than Italy)
- smoking (variable results but appears worse in young people with exudates and older women with proliferative disease)

Surgical treatment

Laser treatment

- Up to 1500–7000 separate burns, of 100–500 μm diameter, each taking about 0.1 s to apply, are needed for panretinal or 'scatter' laser photocoagulation. For oedematous/exudative maculopathy a macula grid may use only 100–200 burns of 100–200 μm diameter separated by 200–400 μm gaps, avoiding the fovea. The ETDRS (Early Treatment Diabetic Retinopathy Study) showed laser therapy was better than no treatment in all visual acuity subgroups, with a 24% blindness rate at 3 years in the non-treated eyes compared to a 12% rate in the treated group.
- Laser therapy is usually performed as 3–4 sessions of outpatient treatment on conscious patients. Topical local anaesthetic drops allow a contact lens to be placed on the cornea and are often all that is needed. In some patients, however, as this procedure may be slightly uncomfortable, a retro-orbital injection (performed through the inside of the lower eyelid) can be given to anaesthetize the eye.
- The laser energy is absorbed by the choroid and the pigment epithelium which lie below the neurosensory layer which also absorbs the energy/heat and is destroyed.
- In patients with severe proliferative retinopathy, pan-retinal photocoagulation reduces visual loss (i.e. an acuity >1/60 or worse) by over 80% while a macula grid reduces visual loss in maculopathy by over 50%.
- Laser treatment aims to prevent further visual loss, especially in maculopathy, not to restore vision, and the distinction must be emphasized to all patients requiring treatment. The benefits from laser therapy currently outweigh the risks, which include accidental burns to the fovea if the eye moves during therapy, a reduction in night vision and, in a small number, interference with visual field severe enough to effect the ability to drive.

Vitrectomy

If the vitreous contains scar tissue, haemorrhage, or any opacity, a vitrectomy to remove it may help restore vision and allows the chance for intraoperative laser treatment or a better view for postoperative laser therapy. It can also help reduce retinal traction and allows retinal reattachment to be performed. A success rate at restoring vision of 70% is seen but the risk of worsening vision, detaching the retina, or worsening lens opacities should also be consider.

Cataract extraction

This is a common procedure with a slightly higher complication rate than in the non-diabetic population. Approximately 15% of patients undergoing a cataract extraction can be expected to have diabetes. A large lens implant should be considered, especially if laser therapy is going to be needed subsequently. Worsening of maculopathy after cataract extraction is also a risk which needs careful monitoring.

Useful addresses

Action for Blind People, 14–16 Verney Road, London SE16 3DZ.
    Tel: 020 7732 8771
Partially Sighted Society, Queen's Road, Doncaster DN1 2NX.
    Tel: 01302 323132
Royal National Institute for the Blind, 224 Great Portland Street, London,
    W1N 6AA. Tel: 020 7388 1266

Further reading

British Multi-Centre Study Group. Photocoagulation for diabetic maculopathy. *Diabetes* 1983; 32: 1010–1016.
Early Treatment Diabetic Retinopathy Study Research Group. *Archives of Ophthalmology* 1985; 103: 1796–1806.

Chapter 4
Diabetic renal disease

Background

Diabetic nephropathy is now a major cause of premature death in patients with all types of diabetes. Approximately 1/6 patients entering most renal replacement programs in developed countries will now have diabetes, at least 50% having type 2 diabetes.

Definition

Diabetic nephropathy is defined as albuminuria (albumin excretion rate >300 mg/24 h, which equates to a 24 h urinary protein >0.5 g) and declining renal function in a patient with known diabetes who does not have a urinary tract infection, heart failure, or any other renal disease. This is usually associated with systemic hypertension, diabetic retinopathy, or neuropathy, and in the absence of these the diagnosis needs to be carefully evaluated.

Epidemiology

Microalbuminuria has a prevalence of 6–60% of patients with type 1 diabetes, after 5–15 years duration of diabetes. Diabetic nephropathy will occur in up to 35% of patients with type 1 diabetes, more commonly in men and in those diagnosed under 15 years of age with a peak incidence approaching 3%/year 16–20 years after onset of diabetes. Of those type 1 patients who develop proteinuria 2/3 will subsequently develop renal failure. In the UK 15% of all deaths in diabetic patients <50 years old are due to nephropathy.

In type 2 patients there are more obvious racial differences, with up to 25% of Caucasians and 50% of Asians expected to develop nephropathy giving a prevalence in a general clinic of 4–33%. The duration of diabetes before development of clinical nephropathy is also often shorter in type 2 than in type 1 patients. This may be due to an initial delay in diagnosis of type 2 diabetes.

Table 4.1 Definitions

Proteinuria	Urinary protein >0.5 g/24 h
Albuminuria	Urinary albumin excretion rate > 300 mg/24 h or >200 µg/min
Microalbuminuria	Urinary albumin excretion rate 30–300 mg/day or 20–200 µg/min

Making the diagnosis

A urine positive on dip testing for protein (i.e. >0.5 mg/L protein or >300 mg/L albumin) suggests diabetic nephropathy. A timed urine collection either overnight or over 24 h will confirm proteinuria or albuminuria, but other causes of proteinuria must be excluded before labelling this diabetic nephropathy. Proteinuria from non-diabetic renal disease occurs in up to 10% of type 1 and 30% of type 2 patients. Urinary tract infections, acute illness, heavy exercise, and cardiac failure are the most common causes to exclude. The absence of hypertension or diabetic retinopathy would also question the diagnosis, and confirmation from a renal biopsy may be required.

If the urine is standard dip test negative for albumin, microalbuminuria should be looked for. The implementation group for the St Vincent Declaration recommend that all patients with negative protein on conventional urinalysis are annually screened for microalbuminuria. A urinary albumin : creatinine ratio >2.5 mg/mmol in men and >3.5 mg/mmol in women or a positive urine dip test (urine albumin >20 μg) should be followed by a timed urine collection repeated three times with at least two abnormal.

Pathology

Although macroscopically there is an increase in kidney size, microscopically there is thickening of the glomerular basement membrane, expansion of glomerular supporting tissues (the mesangium) and fibrotic changes in both efferent and afferent arterioles. If localized this is termed *nodular glomerular sclerosis* (Kimmelsteil–Wilson nodules) and if more widespread, *diffuse glomerular sclerosis*.

The thickened basement membrane initially results in an alteration in its electrical charge but not in pore size, which allows increased passage of albumin into the glomerular ultrafiltrate seen clinically as microalbuminuria.

False positives for microalbuminuria

- exercise
- urinary tract infection
- menstruation
- semen.

Pathogenesis

Hyperglycaemia

As with all microvascular diabetic complications, hyperglycaemia has been implicated in the pathogenesis of diabetic nephropathy via metabolic alterations. The DCCT showed a reduction in the development of microalbuminuria in patients with better glycaemic control, which would support this. The UK PDS showed similar improvements. These metabolic alterations may be due to sorbitol accumulation from the polyol pathway, due to the accumulation of advanced glycation end-products (AGE) or to an as yet unknown mechanism.

AGE have been linked to the extracellular matrix accumulation known to occur in nephropathy. The use of aminoguanidine to block renal AGE accumulation and an associated slowing in the progression of albuminuria and mesangial expansion would support their role in the pathogenesis of nephropathy. The evidence for the polyol pathway's importance comes from aldose reductase inhibitor trials, the results of which are more variable. Ongoing studies (e.g. Action 1 and Action 2 for aminoguanidine) will examine whether any agents are useful clinically.

Haemodynamic alterations

Increased intraglomerular pressures can be associated with elevations in systemic blood pressure (85% of type 1 patients with nephropathy are hypertensive), increased vasoactive hormones (e.g. angiotensin-II, endothelin) or altered levels of specific growth factors (e.g. TGF-β, IGF-I, and VEGF). Hormonal and growth factor alterations have been suggested as important in the initial hyperfiltration phase seen in type 1 patients who progress to nephropathy, and a role for angiotensin-II in the accumulation of extracellular matrix has also been postulated. Whether these changes are secondary to or independent of hyperglycaemia is not certain.

Genetic predisposition

There is an increase in red blood cell sodium–lithium countertransport activity in nephropathic patients and their parents in some populations, and an increased incidence of hypertension in the relatives of diabetic patients with nephropathy. An association between nephropathy and polymorphisms of the ACE gene has also been noted.

Smoking

A consistent link between cigarette smoking and nephropathy has been known for some time, but an aetiological mechanism is not yet known.

Natural history

In 20–40% of type 1 diabetic patients there is initially a period of glomerular hyperfiltration. The first sign of nephropathy, however, is microalbuminuria, usually occurring 5–15 years after the onset of type 1 diabetes but possibly present at the time of diagnosis in type 2 diabetes. Associated with this is often the development of hypertension, a reduction in high-density lipoprotein (HDL)-cholesterol and an increase in LDL-cholesterol and triglycerides.

This progresses to the next stage of frank proteinuria or albuminuria, which has a peak incidence ~17 years after the diagnosis of type 1 diabetes. This is the start of overt nephropathy, as in both type 1 and type 2 patients an approximate 10 ml min^{-1} 1.73 m^{-2} reduction in glomerular filtration rate occurs each year once the albumin excretion rate has reached 300 mg/day, although in some patients the deterioration may be more rapid, and treatment may reduce it. Once serum creatinine concentration reaches 200 μmol/L, a fall of 1 ml/min per month in glomerular filtration rate is then expected. This leads to end-stage renal failure (ESRF) with uraemia and potentially death 7–10 years after onset of albuminuria. A plot of the reciprocal of creatinine against time demonstrates a relatively straight line showing the projected rate of deterioration.

Patients with diabetes and persistent proteinuria/albuminuria have a high mortality, due to cardiovascular disease in 40% of cases. Nephropathy carries a 20–100 times greater mortality than in age-matched diabetic patients without proteinuria.

Risk factors for development of microalbuminuria

- duration of diabetes
- poor long term glycaemic control
- hypertension
- dyslipidaemia
- hyperfiltration
- parents with renal disease.

Treatment

Treatment options for ESRF are either renal dialysis (haemodialysis or ambulatory peritoneal dialysis) or renal transplantation, but life expectancy with either is no better than with some common malignancies. Several other therapies can, however, delay the progression to this stage.

Blood pressure

Controlling hypertension reduces the progression to microalbuminuria and from this to albuminuria and subsequent progression to ESRF. Blood pressure should be reduced to <130/85 mmHg with avoidance of hypotension, although if proteinuria is >1 g/day a better target is <120/75 mmHg. Weight loss, alcohol restriction, and reduced salt intake help, but drugs are usually needed to achieve this.

Studies show benefits from β-blockers, frusemide, hydralazine, and calcium channel blockers, but the ACEIs are currently the preferred first line agent in both microalbuminuric and albuminuric patients as they also have an effect on kidney function independent of their hypotensive action. Several studies suggest, however, that more than one agent will be required to control BP adequately.

Large studies with several ACEIs have confirmed their benefit in hypertensive patients by delaying the progression of microalbuminuria to albuminuria and then to ESRF. There is no documented benefit in treating normotensive patients without microalbuminuria. *Captopril* (50 mg 2× day) for 2 years in type 1 patients with microalbuminuria reduced progression to albuminuria by 68%. *Enalapril* (10 mg daily) given to type 2 patients with microalbuminuria for 5 years reduced progression to albuminuria by 67%. When used for 4 years in type 1 patients with nephropathy, captopril (50 mg 2× day) reduced the risk of death, dialysis, and transplantation by 50% and slowed the reduction in creatinine clearance.

The EUCLID study looked at treating normotensive microalbuminuric type 1 patients. In this study *lisinopril* reduced the albumin excretion rate by nearly 20% compared to placebo but there was a 3 mmHg lower blood pressure in the treatment group. From this it is suggested that normotensive type 1 patients be treated with an ACEIs. An *enalapril* study in normotensive type 2 patients showed similar results.

Glycaemic control

Correction of hyperglycaemia can reverse glomerular basement membrane thickening and mesangial changes. Studies looking at progression to microalbuminuria and subsequent progression to frank albuminuria (e.g. the Steno 1 and II Studies, the KROC Study) also suggest a clinical benefit from improving glycaemic control. In the DCCT tight glycaemic control of type 1 patients was shown to reduce progression to microalbuminuria by 30% and subsequent progression to albuminuria by 54%. Not all trials confirm this (e.g. the Micro-albuminuria Collaborative Study Group Trial and the UK PDS) and not all patients with good control in the above trials gained benefit.

Even so, the current treatment aim is to normalize or significantly reduce HbA1c (<7.2%) while avoiding any weight gain or hypo-glycaemia associated with the increased used of both oral agents and insulin needed to do so.

Dietary protein restriction

High dietary protein can damage the kidney by increasing renal blood flow and intraglomerular pressures in experimental situations. For microalbuminuric type 1 patients reducing dietary animal protein intake in small studies appears to reduce both hyperfiltration and micralbuminuriam, and the benefit in more severe renal impairment is more evident. In type 2 patients the UK PDS showed an initial reduction in microalbuminuria with dietary modification which may in part be related to protein reduction. A dietary protein content <0.8 g/kg is suggested.

Lipid lowering

Although diabetic nephropathy is not shown to reduce the progres-sion of microalbuminuria to albuminuria or renal failure, these patients have a significant dyslipidaemia and a high cardiovascular mortality and require careful lipid monitoring and aggressive treat-ment. The use of aspirin for similar reasons is also advisable.

Further reading

Ahmad J, Siddiqui MA, Ahmad H. Effective postponement of diabetic nephropathy in normotensive type 2 diabetic patients with microalbuminuria. *Diabetes Care* 1997; 20: 1576–1581.

Diabetes Control and Complications Trial Research Group. The effect of intensive treatment of diabetes on the development of microvascular complications of DM. *New England Journal of Medicine* 1993; 329: 304–309.

Diabetes Control and Complications Trial Research Group. Effect of intensive therapy on the development and progression of diabetic nephropathy in the DCCT. *Kidney International* 1995; 42: 1703–1720.

EUCLID Study Group. Randomized placebo-controlled trial of lisinopril in normotensive patients with insulin-dependent diabetes and normoalbuminuria or microalbuminuria. *Lancet* 1997; 349: 1787–1792.

Laffel LMB, McGill JB, Dans DJ on behalf of the North American Microalbuminuria Study Group. The beneficial effect of angiotensin converting enzyme inhibition with captopril on diabetic nephropathy in normotensive IDDM patients with microalbuminuria. *American Journal of Medicine* 1995; 99: 497–504.

Lewis EJ, Hunsicker LG, Bain RP, Rohde RD for the Collaborative Group. The effect of angiotensin converting enzyme inhibition on diabetic nephropathy. *New England Journal of Medicine* 1993; 329: 1456–1462.

Microalbuminuria Captopril Study Group. Captopril reduces the risk of nephropathy in IDDM patients with microalbuminuria. *Diabetologia* 1996; 39: 587–593.

Ravid M, Brosch D, Levi Z *et al.* Use of enalapril to attenuate decline in renal function in normotensive, normalbuminuric patients with type 2 DM. *Annals of Internal Medicine* 1998; 128: 982–988.

UK Prospective Diabetes Study Group. Intensive blood glucose control with sulphonylureas or insulin compared with conventional treatment and risk of complications in patients with type 2 diabetes (UKPDS 33). *Lancet* 1998; 352: 837–853.

UK Prospective Diabetes Study Group. Tight blood pressure control and risk of macrovascular and microvascular complications in type 2 diabetes: UKPDS 38. *BMJ* 1998; 317: 703–713.

UK Prospective Diabetes Study Group. Efficacy of atenolol and captopril in reducing risk of macrovascular and microvascular complications in type 2 diabetes: UKPDS 39. *BMJ* 1998; 317: 713–720.

Chapter 5
Diabetic neuropathy

Involvement of cranial, peripheral, and autonomic nerves may be found in patients with diabetes, and termed diabetic neuropathy; this usually suggests a diffuse, predominantly sensory peripheral neuropathy. The effects on nerve function can be both acute or chronic as well as being transient or permanent. The consequences of neuropathy include:

* neuropathic ulcers, usually on the feet
* Charcot arthropathy
* altered sensation (both pain and increased sensitivity to normal sensation)
* impotence (with autonomic neuropathy).

Pathology

Diabetic neuropathy is one of the microvascular complications of diabetes. Pathologically distal axonal loss occurs with focal demyelination and attempts at nerve regeneration. The vasa nervorum often shows basement membrane thickening, endothelial cell changes, and some occlusion of its lumen. This results in slowing of nerve conduction velocities or a complete loss of nerve function. Both metabolic and vascular changes have been implicated in its aetiology.

Classification of diabetic neuropathies

* sensory neuropathy
  - acute
  - chronic
* autonomic neuropathy
* mononeuropathy
  - entrapment neuropathy
  - external pressure palsies
  - spontaneous mononeuropathy
* proximal motor neuropathy (diabetic amyotrophy)

Pathogenesis

Hyperglycaemia is probably the underlying cause of the histological and functional changes. Several possible mechanisms have been suggested:

- Overloading of the normal pathways for glucose metabolism resulting in increased use of the polyol pathway which leads to increased levels of sorbitol and fructose and decreased levels of myoinositol and glutathione. This may result in more free radical damage and also lowers nitric oxide levels, so altering nerve blood flow. Experimental models using aldose reductase inhibitors which can improve some aspects of diabetic neuropathy add some weight to this theory.

- Possible accumulation of AGE (via non-enzymatic glycation) may also have a role to play, as could the hypercoagulable state and altered blood rheology known to occur in all patients with diabetes. Aminoguanidine, which blocks AGE formation, when used in animal studies can increased both nerve conduction velocities and nerve blood flow in diabetic subjects, strengthening the role of AGE accumulation in this process.

- In the more acute neuropathies, acute ischaemia of the nerves due to vascular abnormalities has been suggested as the cause but again the underlying reason why this should occur is still unclear. Insulin-induced 'neuritis' may occur when insulin therapy is started and blood glucose levels fall.

- Other potential aetiological factors include changes in local growth factor production and oxidative stress.

Further work is needed to clarify the exact role of each of the above mechanisms. In the meantime, studies showing improvements in neuropathy associated with good diabetic control strengthen the argument for the role of hyperglycaemia and offers us one treatment option while we await other therapies.

Peripheral sensorimotor neuropathy

Although hyperglycaemia can alter nerve function and often gives some sensory symptoms at diagnosis, correcting the hyperglycaemia can often resolve these. Chronic sensorimotor neuropathy, on the other hand, is the most common feature of peripheral nerve involvement seen in patients with diabetes. The exact prevalence of diabetic neuropathy varies in most studies because of the different definitions and examination techniques used. For example, sensitive nerve conduction studies can show up to 80% of patients have abnormal results. In more normal practice, however, 20–30% of unselected patients can be expected either to have symptomatic neuropathy or have abnormalities on examination which are clinically significant. But at least 50% of these patients are asymptomatic. This will increase with increasing duration of diabetes, so although 7–8% of type 2 patients may have abnormalities at diagnosis, 50% can be expected to have them 25 years later.

Features

- Usually insidious onset with numbness or paraesthesia, often found on screening rather than as a presenting problem.
- Starts in the toes and on the soles of the feet then spreads up to mid shin level, mostly in a symmetrical fashion. Less often it also involves the fingers and hands.
- Affects all sensory modalities and results in reduced vibration perception thresholds, pinprick, fine touch, and temperature sensations.
- Decreased vibration sensation and absent ankle reflexes are often the first features found. Another risk factor for ulceration is inability to feel a 10 g monofilament.
- Less often the skin is tender/sensitive to touch (hyperaesthesia) or frank pain can occur.
- Painful neuropathy affects up to 5% of a general clinic population. This pain may be sharp, stabbing or burning in nature, and at times very severe.
- There may also be some wasting of the intrinsic muscles of the foot with clawing of the toes.

Mononeuropathies

Peripheral mononeuropathies and cranial mononeuropathies are not uncommon. These may be spontaneous or may be due to entrapment or external pressure. Of the peripheral mono-neuropathies median nerve involvement and carpal tunnel syndrome may be found in up to 10% of patients and require nerve conduction studies and then surgical decompression. Entrapment of the lateral cutaneous nerve of the thigh is also seen more commonly in those with diabetes, giving pain over the lateral aspect of the thigh. Common peroneal nerve involvement causing foot drop and tarsal tunnel syndrome are also recognized but less common.

Cranial mononeuropathies usually occur suddenly and have a good prognosis. Palsies of cranial nerves III and VI are the most common seen, but these are not a common problem in patients with diabetes. In the IIIrd nerve palsy sparing of the pupillary responses is usual. Spontaneous recover is slow over several months and no treatment apart from symptomatic help such as an eye patch is needed. Unlike entrapment neuropathies where decompression may help, no effective treatment is currently available in most of these cases with spontaneous mononeuropathies.

Proximal motor neuropathy (diabetic amyotrophy)

This is an uncommon but disturbing condition to have, mostly affecting men in their 50s with type 2 diabetes. It presents with severe pain and paraesthesia in the upper legs, and is felt as a deep aching pain which may be burning in nature and can keep patients awake at night, put them off eating, and result in marked cachexia. This, with proximal muscle weakness and wasting of the quadriceps in particular, can be very debilitating. The lumbar sacral plexus lower motor neurones are affected and improvement is usually spontaneous over 3–4 months. Before making this diagnosis, however, consider other causes such as malignancies and lumbar disc disease.

Oral antidiabetic agents may play a part in the aetiology of this problem and conversion to insulin therapy is advised, although the anorexia experienced when the pain is severe can make this difficult. Although recovery happens over a few months only 50% recover fully, but no other treatment is currently known to improve on this.

Examination

* Mandatory at diagnosis and at least yearly in all asymptomatic patients.
* Test vibration, fine touch (with a 10 g monofilament), and reflexes as a minimum. Using a neurothesiometer or biosthesiometer gives a more quantitative measure of vibration than a 128 Hz tuning fork. Inability to feel the vibrating head at >25 V in the toes is associated with a significant risk of neuropathic ulceration and should be considered a sign of 'at risk' feet.

Differential diagnoses

* uraemia
* vitamin B_{12} deficiency
* infections (e.g. HIV and leprosy)
* toxins (e.g. alcohol, lead, mercury)
* malignancy.

Treatment

* *For all patients* Review by a chiropodist and if indicated an orthotist to give education on foot care and suitable footwear is advised. If followed by regular chiropody review this can help prevent some problems developing.
* *Asymptomatic patients* No drugs are yet available, but aldose reductase inhibitors such as *tolrestat* are advocated for this indication by some.
* *Painful neuropathy* Initially try capsaicin 0.075% topically to the affected area, being careful to avoid normal skin because this chili pepper extract, which depletes sensory nerve terminals of substance P, can be uncomfortable when applied to normal skin. It can take several weeks to be effective and may induce tingling and so worsening of symptoms initially. In some patients simple analgesics such as *paracetamol* or opiates such as *tramadol* have been shown to help. In more severe cases tricyclic antidepressants are the first line treatment of choice with *imipramine* 20–100 mg at night being less sedative than *amitriptyline* 25–75 mg. Although newer agents such as *carbamazepine*, *phenytoin*, and *paroxetine* have less anticholinergic effects, they are also not as effective and are therefore used as second line, although recent data for *gabapentin* may buck this trend. If the pain is severe and like an electric shock, anticonvulsants such as *carbamazepine* and *phenytoin* may however be more effective.
* *Hyperaesthesia* Occlusive dressings such as Opsite may prove helpful. For more severe pain, oral agents are needed.

General treatments

Specific treatments for each form of neuropathy have been discussed above, but there is some evidence for more general therapies.

• Poor diabetic control appears to be associated with worsening neuropathy and improving glycaemic control is advocated in any patient, especially if neuropathy is present.

• The use of evening primrose oil in rats and preliminary human studies suggests this may improve some aspects of diabetic neuropathy. The mechanism by which this works is not certain but it does increase production of cyclo-oxygenase-mediated prostanoids such as prostacyclin which could act as a vasodilator and so improve nerve blood supply.

• Other more specific vasodilators have also been examined, with α blockers and ACEIs showing particularly useful results in experimental settings.

• Polyol pathway inhibition with aldose reductase inhibitors and non-enzymatic glycation inhibition with agents such as aminoguanidine are also being examined.

• An alternative approach is not to try to improve the underlying problem but to alter the body's response to it. Nerve growth factor (NGF) and IGF-I have been examined for their ability to cause nerve regeneration and growth, and NGF in particular looks potentially very interesting. Other such agents are also under investigation.

Autonomic neuropathy

The commonest effect of autonomic neuropathy is erectile dysfunction which affects 40% of men with diabetes. Only a small number develop the severe gastrointestinal and bladder dysfunction. The recent interest in *sildenafil* has highlighted this. Abnormal autonomic function tests can be expected in 20–40% of a general diabetic clinic population. The increased problems during surgery from cardiac involvement should be remembered.

Clinical features

- impotence
- postural hypotension (giving dizziness and syncope in up to 12%)
- resting tachycardia or fixed heart rate/loss of sinus arrhythmia (in up to 20%)
- gustatory sweating (sweating after tasting food)
- dysphagia with delayed gastric emptying, nausea/vomiting
- constipation/diarrhoea
- urinary retention/overflow incontinence
- anhidrosis (absent sweating on the feet is especially problematic as it increases the risk of ulceration)
- abnormal pupillary reflexes.

Assessment

At least annually check:

- lying and standing BP (measure systolic BP 2 min after standing; normal is <10 mmHg drop, > 30 mmHg is abnormal)
- pupillary responses to light.

Other less commonly performed tests to consider if the diagnosis is uncertain or in high risk patients include:

- *Loss of sinus arrhythmia* Measure inspiratory and expiratory heart rates after 5 s of each (<10 beats/min difference is abnormal, >15 is normal).
- *Loss of heart rate response to Valsalva manoeuvre* Look at the ratio of the shortest R-R interval during forced expiration against a closed glottis compared to the longest R-R interval after it (<1.2 is abnormal).
- *Blood pressure response to sustained hand grip* Diastolic blood pressure prior to the test is compared to diastolic blood pressure after

5 min of sustaining a grip equivalent to 30% of maximal grip. A diastolic BP rise >16 mmHg is normal, <10 mmHg is abnormal. A rolled up blood pressure cuff to achieve the required hand grip may be used.

- For *gastric symptoms* consider a radioisotope test meal to look for delayed gastric emptying.

Treatment

This is based on the specific symptom and is usually symptomatic only. In all patients improvement in diabetic control is advocated in case any of it is reversible, but this is not usually very helpful or effective.

Postural hypotension

- May be exacerbated by drugs such as diuretics, vasodilators, and tricyclic antidepressants.
- Mechanical measures such as sleeping with the head elevated and wearing support stockings may help.
- Ensure an adequate salt intake.
- *Fludrocortisone* 50 μg once daily initially and increased as required up to 400 μg may be helpful, but beware of hypertension or oedema.
- *Desmopressin* and *octreotide* have also been used.

Impotence

Libido is not normally affected and pain is also unusual, so look for hypogonadism and Peyronie's if they are present. Autonomic neuropathy is the likely cause but many drugs, especially thiazides and β-blockers, can also cause it, as can alcohol, tobacco, cannabis, and stress. These should be assessed by direct questioning. Examination should include:

- genitalia and secondary sexual characteristics
- peripheral pulses (as vascular insufficiency may play a part)
- lower limb reflexes and vibration thresholds (to confirm that neuropathy is present).

  Biochemical screening should at least include:

- prolactin
- testosterone
- gonadotrophins (LH/FSH).

  Exacerbating factors such as alcohol and antihypertensive drugs should be modified. The main therapies are:

- *sildenafil* (start at 25–50 mg, increase to 100 mg if needed)

- intraurethral *alprostadil* (start at 125 µg, increase to 250 or 500 *µ*g if needed)
- intracavernosal *alprostadil* (trial dose is 2.5 *µ*g, treatment is 5–40 *µ*g)
- vacuum devices.

None of these is ideal. Sildenafil, although an oral therapy, is effective in only 60% of those with diabetes and is contraindicated with severe heart disease and those on nitrates, which rules many out.

Gastroparesis

Delayed gastric emptying can cause recurrent hypoglycaemic episodes. Promotilic agents can also help. Treatment options:

- *cisapride* (10 mg pre-meals/3–4 × day) – now withdrawn in the UK
- *metoclopramide* (5–10 mg pre-meals/3 × day)
- *domperidone* (10–20 mg pre-meals)
- *erythromycin* (acts as a motilin agonist to increase gastric emptying but may make patients feel nauseated so of limited use)
- surgery (gastric drainage procedures should not be undertaken lightly).

Large bowel involvement

Constipation is treated with standard bulking and softening laxatives. The episodic diarrhoea is more troublesome, and treatment for this may include:

- *loperamide* (2 mg 4× day) or codeine phosphate (30 mg 4× day)
- antibiotics in case of bacterial overgrowth, such as *erythromycin* 250 mg 4× day for 7 days, or tetracycline 250 mg 2× day for 7 days
- other agents such as *clonidine* and *ondansetron* have also shown some benefit.

Neuropathic bladder

Sacral nerve involvement can cause bladder abnormalities with reduced sensations of bladder fullness and increased residual volume after micturition. Regular toileting initially may help but intermittent self-catheterization or a long-term catheter may be required.

Anhidrosis

Dry feet can cause cracks in the skin and act as a site for infection. Emollient creams may help prevent this.

Further reading

Boulton AJM, Gries FA, Jervell LA. Guidelines for the diagnosis and outpatient management of diabetic peripheral neuropathy. *Diabetic Medicine* 1998; 15(6): 508–514.

Chapter 6
Macrovascular disease

People with diabetes have a significantly greater risk of coronary heart disease, cerebrovascular disease, and peripheral vascular disease than the non-diabetic population. Most people with diabetes will die from one of these (75% of patients with Type 2).

Epidemiology

The exact prevalence and incidence of macrovascular disease and its outcomes will vary depending on the age, sex, and ethnic mix of the patients being assessed. In general cardiovascular disease accounts for 75% of deaths in type 2 patients and 35% in type 1 patients. Although the atheroma seen is histologically the same as in a non-diabetic population, it tends to be more diffuse and progresses more rapidly. It also occurs at an earlier age and affects both sexes equally: women therefore seem to lose their natural premenopausal advantage.

- Overall peripheral vascular disease occurs in up to 10% of patients and they have up to 15-fold greater risk of needing a non-traumatic amputation than the non-diabetic population.
- Thromboembolic cerebrovascular events occurs in up to 8%, which is a 2–4-fold increased risk compared to the non-diabetic population and accounts for 15% of deaths in type 2 patients.
- The risk of having a myocardial infarction is also increased 2–4 times. Women seem particularly at risk of cardiovascular disease compared to the non-diabetic population.

Patients with type 1 diabetes have half the rate of coronary heart disease, 1/3 the rate of cerebrovascular disease, and 2/3 the rate of peripheral vascular disease compared to type 2 patients, but their rate of all these is greater than that for the non-diabetic population. Men and women are equally affected, with the incidence rates for ischaemic heart disease about 6 times that of both cerebrovascular and peripheral vascular disease.

Secondary prevention

- stop smoking
- aspirin
- β-blockers
- lipid lowering drugs.

Pathogenesis

Atherosclerosis has a well known set of risk factors, such as smoking and family history, all of which still apply in a diabetic population. Some factors, however, are more common in those with diabetes and may also confer a greater risk to the diabetic population. These include:

- *Glycaemic control* In type 1 patients worsening hyperglycaemia is said to relate to the degree of disease present. In type 2 patients this association is less clear cut, although the UKPDS does suggest this is also the case as better glycaemic control was associated with a trend for fewer myocardial infarctions.

- *Hypertension* More common in both type 1 and type 2 patients and results in vascular endothelial injury so predisposing to atheroma formation. The UKPDS suggests blood pressure control is a more important individual risk factor than glycaemic control.

- *Hyperlipidaemia* Common: e.g. hyperinsulinaemia in insulin-resistant type 2 patients causes reduced HDL-cholesterol, elevated triglycerides (and VLDL), and smaller denser and therefore more atherogenic LDL-cholesterol.

- *Obesity* An independent risk factor, more common in type 2 patients. Central obesity in particular is more atherogenic.

- *Insulin resistance* or elevated circulating insulin/proinsulin-like molecule levels are known to increase the risk of atherosclerosis in both diabetic and non-diabetic populations. This may be linked to impaired endothelial function.

- *Altered coagulability* Circulating fibrinogen, platelet activator inhibitor (PAI)-1 and von Willebrand factor levels are increased and platelets are less deformable. This may be more prothrombotic, but the exact significance remains uncertain.

The UKPDS has shown the major risk factors for coronary heart disease in type 2 patients to be elevated LDL-cholesterol, decreased HDL-cholesterol, hypertension, hyperglycaemia, and smoking. Exactly why these risk factors are commonly seen/linked in the same patient, particularly type 2 diabetic patients, is uncertain. Several hypotheses have been put forward, but none as yet explains them all adequately. However, each suggests an element of genetic susceptibility mixed with environmental effects. A genetic predisposition to insulin resistance, for example, may combine with poor intrauterine nutrition to produce a low birthweight infant with a susceptibility to vascular disease and diabetes later in life. But other factors must be involved. as not all those who later develop diabetes and vascular disease were small at birth.

Lipid abnormalities found in patients with diabetes

Hyperlipidaemia in a patient with diabetes, at any level of cholesterol, is associated with a greater risk of macrovascular disease than in a non-diabetic population. Patients with diabetes may have altered activity of insulin-dependent enzymes such as lipoprotein lipase which results in delayed systemic clearance of certain lipids. This, combined with altered hepatic production of apoprotein-B containing lipoproteins, gives a more atherogenic profile.

Usual findings are of increased triglyceride containing lipoproteins, chylomicrons, and VLDL. Although more common in the insulin-resistant type 2 patients this can also be seen in type 1 patients as can a low HDL-cholesterol (HDL_2 especially). Other atherogenic changes include a tendency to develop small dense LDL cholesterol particles and a greater tendency to oxidative damage which renders them even more atherogenic. Lipoprotein (Lpa) levels are also often raised.

Even so, other common primary causes of hyperlipidaemia, such as familial hypercholesterolaemia or familial combined hyperlipidaemia, should not be missed. Screening for secondary causes of hyperlipidaemia such as hypothyroidism or drug induced (alcohol, thiazides, and β blockers in particular) is also strongly advised.

Management

In all patients the first treatment is dietary modification. In a patient who is actually following a good diabetic diet, however, there is often not much room for improvement.

Other standard advice should also be given:

- stop smoking (reduces risk of death by about 50% over a 15 year period)
- reduce weight if overweight/obese
- increase physical activity.

While the reductions in mortality, re-infarction, and stroke in the major lipid lowering trials such as the 4S study (Scandinavian Simvastatin Survival Study), CARE (Cholesterol and Recurrent Events Trial), LIPID (Long-term Intervention with Pravastatin in Ischaemic Disease), and WOSCOPS (West of Scotland Coronary Prevention Study) are all very impressive, the diabetic subgroups show as good if not better reductions although the numbers in each were relatively small. In 4S, for example, the simvastatin-treated diabetic subgroup (4.5% of those in the study) had a 23% rate of major coronary events

Table 6.1 Lipid reduction studies

	4S	WOSCOP	CARE	LIPID
Type of study	Secondary prevention of CHD	Primary prevention of CHD	Secondary prevention of CHD	Secondary prevention of CHD
Duration of study (years)	6	5	5	6
Number studied	4444	6595	4159	9014
Mean total cholesterol (mmol/L) (range)	6.8 (5.5–8.0)	7.0 (>6.5)	5.4 (<6.2)	(4.0–7.0)
Age range (years)	35–70	45–64	21–75	31–75
% men	81	100	86	83
% with diabetes	4.5	1	17	8.6
Treatment	Simvastatin 20–40 mg daily	Pravastatin 40 mg daily	Pravastatin 40 mg daily	Pravastatin 40 mg daily
Event reduction for major coronary events	34% for non-diabetics 55% for diabetics	31% overall	23% for non-diabetics 25% for diabetics	23% overall

compared to 45% in the diabetic placebo group, while the non-diabetic simvastatin group had 19% and the placebo non-diabetic group had 27%. On the basis of this it is suggested that if 100 patients with diabetes who have angina or are post myocardial infarction are treated with simvastatin for 6 years, 24 of the 46 expected coronary deaths and non-fatal myocardial infarctions can be prevented. Ongoing lipid lowering trials including larger numbers with diabetes such as CARDS (Collaborative Atorvastatin Diabetes Study) and ASPEN (Atorvastatin Study for the Prevention of Endpoints in Non-insulin dependent diabetes) will help to clarify this further.

Once the above lifestyle measures have been implemented, consider the need for drug therapy. The Sheffield tables, New Zealand tables or the Joint British Societies Coronary Risk Predicion Chart should be used to determine risk in primary prevention. In a diabetic patient a total cholesterol : HDL-cholesterol ratio is preferable to using total cholesterol alone, especially in women. Also, while a 3% risk cut-off is advocated by many, the use of a 1.5–2% level in higher risk groups such as the diabetic population is not without support. Remember that a fit patient with diabetes has a similar risk when compared to a non- diabetic of the same age and sex who has also had a coronary event. In those with known coronary heart disease, cerebrovascular or peripheral vascular disease use the 1997 Standing Medical Advisory Committee guidelines for statins in secondary prevention. These suggest, following a trial of dietary modification:

- Treat a total cholesterol >4.8 mmol/L or an LDL-cholesterol >3.3 mmol/L using pharmacological agents such as statins.
- The treatment aim is a total cholesterol <4.5 and an LDL of <2.6 mmol/L.

Lower targets for each are advocated by many, especially for those patients post coronary artery bypass grafting or post angioplasty. Triglycerides should be brought <1.5 mmol/L, as above this athero-genic lipoprotein changes are said to occur.

In those with mixed hyperlipidaemia, consider a fibrate or a statin licenced for this indication. A fibrate will reduce triglycerides by 30–40% and LDL-cholesterol by 20% while a statin would reduce triglycerides slightly less (10–15%) and LDL-cholesterol slightly more (25–35%). Fibrates also alter the LDL-cholesterol to its less athero-genic form. The choice of agent must be tailored to the individual patient. For hypercholesterolaemia alone a statin is first choice, as in the non-diabetic patient, and in severely resistant patients combination therapy with statins, fibrates, and less often resins may be required.

Treatment aims for lipids

Primary prevention
- Treat if risk table analysis gives a >3% risk per year.

Secondary prevention
Following failure of diet treat:
- total cholesterol >4.8 mmol/L to <4.5 mmol/L (or <4.0 post CABG/angioplasty)
- LDL cholesterol >3.3 mmol/L to <2.6 mmol/L
- aim to have triglycerides <1.5 mmol/L.

Investigations
Take a full history and carefully examine the patient. In all patients then check:
- dip test urine for protein
- serum urea, electrolytes, and creatinine (and creatinine clearance if creatinine is raised)
- fasting lipids
- ECG (for left ventricular hypertrophy and signs of ischaemia).

Also consider:
- the need for a chest radiograph for signs of heart failure/cardiomegaly
- an echocardiogram
- cortisol + dexamethasone suppression test
- catecholamines
- renin/aldosterone.

Hypertension

Epidemiology

Hypertension is twice as common in the diabetic population as in the non-diabetic population, and standard ethnic differences in the prevalence of hypertension still hold true. It is known that hypertension worsens the severity of and increases the risk of developing both microvascular and macrovascular disease. Using a cut-off of >160/90 mmHg, hypertension occurs in:

- 10–30% of patients with type 1 diabetes
- 20–30% of microalbuminuric type 1 patients
- 80–90% of macroalbuminuric type 1 patients
- 30–50% of Caucasians with type 2 diabetes.

Using the UKPDS suggested target of 140/80, hypertension is even more common.

Pathogenesis

- *Type 1 patients* Hypertension is strongly associated with diabetic nephropathy and microalbuminuria and occurs at an earlier stage than that seen in many other causes of renal disease. This may inpart be linked to a genetic predisposition also giving increased activity in red blood cell sodium–lithium counter-transport activity which leads to increased peripheral vascular resistance. Insulin may also have a suppressive effect on renin release, so giving hyporeninaemic hypoaldosteronism.

- *Type 2 patients* Hypertension is associated with insulin resistance and hyperinsulinaemia; again, this may be genetically mediated. Hyperinsulinaemia can directly cause hypertension by increasing sympathetic nervous system activity, increasing proximal tubule sodium resorption, and stimulating vascular smooth muscle cell proliferation. Hyperglycaemia also has an antinatiuretic effect and with hyperinsulinaemia leading to hypokalaemia which results in both glucose and sodium reabsorption being increased all increases the potential for hypertension.

Management

Treatment aim

The current recommendation is for all patients with diabetes to have a blood pressure <140/80 mmHg. The hypertension study in the UKPDS highlights the benefits for type 2 patients of such a treatment

Management of acute myocardial infarction

Patients with diabetes are more likely to have a myocardial infarction and more likely to die from it than the non-diabetic population. This may be due to a greater likelihood of myocardial pump failure. Several studies highlight this:

Trial and outcome examined	Non-diabetic subgroup	Diabetic subgroup
ISSI-2		
Non-streptokinase 4 year mortality	27%	41%
GUSTO		
In-hospital mortality	6.2%	10.6%
GISSI-2		
Re-infarction rates	14%	30%

Up to 20–40% of patients admitted to hospital with a myocardial infarction will have hyperglycaemia, many of whom will not have previously diagnosed diabetes.

As in the non-diabetic population, streptokinase and aspirin have proven benefits. The previous contraindication for thrombolysis in those with proliferative diabetic retinopathy has been questioned by many. Tight glycaemic control (blood glucose 7–10 mmol/L) using i/v glucose and insulin for at least 24 h followed by s/c insulin, as used in the DIGAMI study, also has benefits. In this study, patients with an admission blood glucose >11.0 mmol/L who were treated with this regimen had a 7.5% absolute risk reduction in mortality at 1 year and an 11% risk reduction at 3.5 years compared to the control group (i.e. 33% mortality with treatment vs 44% in controls at 3.5 years). This equates to 1 life saved for every 9 treated with this regimen. The exact reason for this is unclear.

- It is suggested that all patients with a blood glucose >11 mmol/L benefit from such treatment whether previously known to have diabetes or not. Using an admission HbA1c to detect those with undiagnosed or stress-related hyperglycaemia can be useful, but should not result in withholding the acute treatment of this hyperglycaemia in such patients. It may, however, help to identify those who may be troubled by hypoglycaemia and may not therefore be suitable for s/c insulin or sulfonylureas in the intermediate or long term.

- Using ACEIs early after myocardial infarction gives a 0.5% absolute risk reduction in 30 day mortality and a 4–8% risk reduction over 15–50 months in a general population. Analysis of the diabetic subgroup in the GISSI-3 study showed a 30% reduction in 6 week mortality for the diabetics (8.7% vs 12.4%) compared to a 5% reduction for non-diabetics. In view of the greater proportion of diabetics with poor left ventricular function after myocardial infarction compared to the non-diabetic population, this difference is very important.

level on mortality, diabetes related end-points, and microvascular end-points. In this a 10/5 mmHg difference in blood pressure was associated with a 34% risk reduction in macrovascular end-points, a 37% risk reduction in microvascular end-points, and a 44% risk reduction in stroke. The recent Hypertension Optimum Treatment (HOT) study again suggests a target of <140/80 mmHg although in those who already have significant end-organ damage a lower target is advocated by some (<130/80).

Predisposing conditions
Other conditions which can cause both hypertension and hyperglycaemia should be considered, e.g. Cushing's syndrome, acromegaly, and phaeochromocytoma (see relevant sections).

End-organ damage
Look for evidence of end-organ damage (eyes, heart, kidneys, and peripheral vascular tree in particular).

Assessment of cardiac risk factors
Look for associated risk factors for coronary heart disease.

Treatment

General
Once this initial assessment is complete, modify other risk factors such as glycaemic control, smoking, and dyslipidaemia. Then look at:
- weight reduction if obese
- reduced salt intake (<6 g/day)
- reduced alcohol intake (<21 units/week in men,<14 in women)
- exercise (20–40 min of moderate exertion 3–5 times/week).

Pharmacological
After this, start drug therapy for the hypertension. Most agents currently available will drop systolic blood pressure by no more than 20 mmHg at most. Remember that in the UKPDS blood pressure study, 1/3 of those achieving the tight blood pressure targets we are now aiming for required three or more drugs to do so.
- In the presence of microalbuminuria or frank proteinuria, always consider an ACEI first line.
- In Afro-Caribbean diabetics a diuretic may also be needed to improve the efficacy of the ACEI as these and ß-blockers are less effective than calcium channel blockers and diuretics in these patients.
- Although many studies suggest the superiority of the ACEI the UKPDS did not confirm any difference between captopril and

atenolol, so if urinalysis is clear other agents such as loop or thiazide diuretics, β-blockers, and calcium channel blockers are also often used first line.

- These agents are again used second line but also consider angiotensin-II receptor blockers and α-blockers, both of which are probably under-used.
- Several agents, such as high dose thiazides and β-blockers, can, however, worsen diabetic control, mask hypoglycaemia, and exacerbate dyslipidaemia so tailor the drugs chosen to each patient.
- In those with angina a β-blocker has added benefits
- In those with peripheral vascular disease vasodilators such as the calcium channel blockers and α-blockers are beneficial.

The ongoing Antihypertensive and Lipid Lowering Treatment to Prevent Heart Attack Trial (ALLHAT), which includes a large diabetic cohort, should give further help when choosing which agent to start with.

Further reading

Hanssen L, Zanchetti A, Carruthers SG *et al.* Effects of intensive blood pressure lowering and low dose aspirin in patients with hypertension: principal results of the Hypertension Optimum Treatment (HOT) randomised trial. *Lancet* 1998; 351: 1755–1762.

Malmberg K for the DIGAMI (DM, Insulin Glucose Infusion in Acute Myocardial) study group. Prospective randomized study of intensive insulin treatment on long term survival after acute myocardial infarction in patients with DM. *BMJ* 1997; 314: 1512–1515.

Pyorala K, Pedersen TR, Kjekshus J *et al.* Cholesterol lowering with simvastatin improves prognosis of diabetic patients with coronary heart disease. *Diabetes Care* 1997; 20: 614–620.

UKPDS Group. Tight blood pressure control and risk of macrovascular and microvascular complications in type 2 diabetes: UKPDS 38. *BMJ* 1998; 317: 703–713.

UKPDS Group. Efficacy of atenolol and captopril in reducing the risk of macrovascular and microvascular complications in type 2 diabetes: UKPDS 39. *BMJ* 1998; 317: 713–720.

Zuanetti G *et al.* Effect of the ACE inhibitor lisinopril in diabetic patients with acute myocardial infarction. Data from GISSI-3 Study. *Circulation* 1997; 96: 4239–4245.

Chapter 7
Diabetic foot

Risk factors for foot ulcer development

Several features/factors are thought to predispose to ulcer formation, and awareness of these may highlight 'at risk' patients for education and other preventive strategies. These ulcers can occur anywhere on the foot, but the tips of claw/hammer toes and over the metatarsal heads are the most frequent sites. The risk factors/features include:

- *Peripheral neuropathy* (seen in up to 80% of diabetic patients with foot ulcers) reduces awareness of pain and trauma caused by footwear and foreign bodies in shoes. Look for reduced mono-filament sensation (e.g. reduced to a 10 g monofilament) and reduced vibration perception thresholds (e.g. reduced sensation to a 128 Hz tuning fork for <10 s or >25 V with a biosthesiometer), suggesting at risk feet.

- *Autonomic neuropathy* leading to anhidrosis can dry out the skin and cause it to crack, so allowing a portal of entry for infection. These feet are often warm and dry with distended veins.

- *Motor neuropathy* can result in altered foot muscle tone, wasting of small muscles, raising of the medial longitudinal arch, and clawing of the toes which can put more pressure through the metatarsal heads and heels so predisposing to callus and ulcer formation. Electrophysiology can help examine this, but is too invasive for widespread routine use.

- *Peripheral vascular disease* (seen in up to 10% of patients) and *microvascular circulatory disease* leads to local ischaemia, increasing the potential for ulcer formation and can delay wound healing when ulceration occurs. Always examine peripheral pulses and consider doppler studies if abnormal. An ankle : brachial artery ratio of >1.1 suggests arterial disease.

- *Duration of diabetes* relates to the presence of the above factors but is often quoted as an independent risk factor, as is increasing age. But type 2 diabetes may be present and undiagnosed for some time.

- The presence of *other microvascular complications* such as nephro-pathy and retinopathy is also a risk factor for foot ulcer develop-ment.

- *Previous ulceration* is another important risk factor, and anyone with previous problems deserves very careful monitoring/follow up.

Table 7.1 Epidemiology of foot ulceration in the UK

Prevalence of foot ulceration	5–10%
Number of people with diabetes developing foot ulcers	14 000–42 000
Proportion of people with diabetes undergoing lower limb amputation	1%
Number of people with diabetes undergoing lower limb amputation per year	2000
Annual NHS expenditure on diabetes foot-related care	£13 million

Table 7.2 Clinical features of diabetic feet

Neuropathic feet	Ischaemic feet
Warm	Cold/cool
Dry skin	Atrophic/often hairless
Palpable foot pulses	No palpable foot pulses
No discomfort with ulcer	More often tender/painful
Callus present	Claudication/Rest pain
	Skin blanches on elevation and reddens on dependency

Table 7.3 Wagner's classification of diabetic foot lesions

Grade 0	High risk foot, no ulceration present
Grade 1	Superficial ulcer, not infected
Grade 2	Deep ulcer with or without cellulitis but no abscess or bone involvement
Grade 3	Deep ulcer with bone involvement or abscess formation
Grade 4	Localized gangrene (toe, forefoot, heel)
Grade 5	Gangrene of the whole foot

From Wagner (1983).

- *Lack of diabetes monitoring* and lack of previous examinations of the feet are also recognized risk factors.
- *Mechanical, chemical or thermal trauma/injury* are often the predisposing factor, and any profession or pastime that increases the risk of these is a risk factor.

Treatment

This is a multidisciplinary problem requiring collaboration between interested diabetologists, diabetes nurse specialists, chiropodists, orthotists, vascular surgeons, plastic surgeons, and occasionally orthopaedic surgeons. Treatment is aimed at several distinct areas, namely:

* at-risk feet with no current ulceration
* treating existing ulcers
* treating infected ulcers
* treating osteomyelitis
* treating vascular insufficiency.

At-risk feet with no current ulceration

When at-risk feet are identified in any patient with diabetes, standard advice should be given and this will need to be repeated/reinforced regularly. This advice would usually include:

* General advice on nail care, hygiene and care with footwear – often best from the chiropodist.
* Reinforce the need for regular daily examination of the feet by the patient or carer.
* Consider regular chiropody review as well as self-monitoring. Also reinforce the need for more urgent review if the patient discovers problems.
* Consider the need for modification of footwear or special footwear if there are abnormalities with foot posture or problems with pressure loading on certain parts of the foot. Padded socks can also reduce trauma. Advise the patient to examine shoes before putting them on, wear lace-ups or shoes with lots of room for the toes and avoid ill-fitting fashion shoes. In some people protective toecaps can prove very useful.
* Avoid walking barefoot.

At the moment no other therapy is advocated in this group of patients, but, as discussed in the neuropathy section, good diabetic control is important and other agents may be useful in the future such as aldose reductase inhibitors, inhibitors of non-enzymatic glycation, and various growth factors.

Existing ulcers

All ulcers should be considered deep and involving bone until proved otherwise. Also:

The Charcot foot

Epidemiology
This is a relatively rare complication of diabetes: an average district general hospital clinic will have 3–10 patients with this problem.

Pathogenesis
It is suggested that blood flow increases due to sympathetic nerve loss. This causes osteoclast activity and bone turnover to increase, so making the bones of the foot more susceptible to damage. Even minor trauma can therefore result in destructive changes in this susceptible bone.

Clinical features
The most likely site is the tarsal–metatarsal region or the metatarsophalangeal joints. Initially it gives a warm/hot, swollen, and often uncomfortable foot, which may be indistinguishable from cellulitis and gout. Peripheral pulses are invariably present and peripheral neuropathy is evident clinically.

Plain radiographs will be normal initially and later show fractures with osteolysis and joint reorganization with subluxation of the metatarsophalangeal joints and dislocation of the large joints of the foot. Isotope scans with technetium are abnormal from early on, but differentiation form infective or other inflammatory causes can be difficult. MRI scanning may prove more useful for this in the future as may [111]indium-labelled white cell studies if infection is suspected.

Eventually, in the untreated patient, two classic deformities are seen:

- a 'rocker bottom' deformity due to displacement and subluxation of the tarsus downwards
- medial convexity due to displacement of the talonavicular joint or tarsometatarsal dislocation.

Management
If diagnosed early, immobilization may help prevent joint destruction. Exactly how best to do this is not agreed but using a non-walking plaster cast or an Aircast type of boot is needed for at least 2–3 months while bone repair/remodelling is going on. Some advocate immobilization for anything up to a year. The recent use of bisphosphates to speed this up by reducing osteoclast activity is interesting and already under further evaluation.

- *Optimize diabetic control*.
- *Reduction of oedema* is important to aid healing.
- *Regular debridement* of callus and dead tissue/skin is important for both neuropathic and ischaemic ulcers. Debridement is usually best with a scalpel and forceps although chemical agents (such as *Varidase*, which contains streptokinase) can occasionally help. But, as these agents can also damage healthy tissue, use under careful supervision. More recently the use of sterile maggots has been shown to be effective. After debridement apply dressings but change these regularly. Be careful that tight dressings do not impair a poor circulation further and that thick dressings or quantities of sticky tape to hold them on do not cause their own skin trauma or pressure effects.
- *Infection control* Infection may be localized but any evidence of deeper infection or sinus formation raises the possibility of osteomyelitis. Systemic symptoms may be minimal as may pain/tenderness so be suspicious of more severe infection than you can see in everyone. The organisms may be ordinary skin commensals given a port of entry but send swabs for culture and think of *Staphylococcus aureus* or streptococci as likely organisms.

  If a sinus is present, probe it and if down to bone assume there is osteomyelitis. Culture anything you get out. Plain radiographs may show bone erosion or destruction with osteomyelitis; radioisotope scans using technetium can show increased uptake with both infection and Charcot arthropathy. The use of MRI scanning can be useful to differentiate in this situation.

  If infection is present use triple therapy with *flucloxacillin* (500 mg 4× daily), *ampicillin/amoxicillin* (500 mg 3× daily) and *metronidazole* (200 mg 3× daily) or consider using *amoxicillin/clavulanic acid* (250/125 mg 3× daily) or *ciprofloxacin* (500–750 mg 2× daily) and *clindamycin* (300–450 mg 2× daily) depending on the organisms grown and patient tolerability. This will need to be i/v/rectal initially if the infection is severe and for the deeper infections several months of therapy may be needed. If osteomyelitis is present consider using *ciprofloxacin* or *sodium fusidate* which have better bone penetration and again use for several months.

  In some patients this approach fails to control osteomyelitis adequately and resection/amputation is required, so regular liaison with an interested surgeon is imperative.

- *Reducing trauma* and *pressure relief* in neuropathic ulcers Padded socks can reduce sheer stress and trauma. Suitable shoes and insoles can help to relieve pressure to allow healing to occur as long as unnecessary walking is minimized. If this is not enough a pneumatic boot/Aircast boot or a total contact cast may be needed. These allow the patient to be mobile but take the weight away from the ulcerated area or foot and put all the weight/pressure through to the calf instead. The involvement of both chiropodists and orthotists is therefore essential.

• *Revascularization* Always consider coexistent vascular disease in a neuropathic foot or predominantly ischaemic ulcers/feet. Vascular bypass grafting/reconstruction or angioplasty can give excellent results with a 70–95% limb salvage rate often quoted. The improved blood supply will also help healing of existing ulcers and may negate the need for amputation or allow the area requiring resection to be minimized. If vascular intervention is unsuccessful or not possible then amputation is required, preferably as a below-knee procedure to give a better mobilization potential postoperatively.

Further reading

Boulton AJM. Foot problems in patients with DM. Chapter 58 in Williams G, Pickup JC (ed.), *Textbook of Diabetes*, 2nd edn, 1997. Oxford: Blackwell Science.

Management of Diabetic Foot Disease. A National Clinical Guideline recommended for use in Scotland by the Scottish Intercollegiate Network (SIGN). 1997 (available from SIGN Secretariat, 9 Queen Street, Edinburgh, EH2 1JQ).

Wagner FW. Algorithms of diabetic foot care. In: Levin ME, O'Neil LW, eds. *The Diabetic Foot*, 2nd edn. St Louis: Mosby Yearbook, 1983: 291–302.

Chapter 8
Diabetes and pregnancy

Background

2–4/1000 women who become pregnant have previously known diabetes, and 2–3% of pregnant women have a diagnosis of gestational diabetes made during their pregnancy. In both cases there are risks both to the mother and the foetus, with an historical foetal abnormality rate of up to 30% or 12 times that of the background population often being quoted.

Risks

Foetal

With greater emphasis on improving glycaemic control, a 2.5–3-fold increased congenital malformation rate in mothers with previously known diabetes and a 1.8-fold increase in those without, compared to the non-diabetic population, is more realistic now. Cardiac, renal, and neural tube defects occur, particularly sacral agenesis. Hyperglycaemia in the first 8 weeks of foetal life, during organogenesis, is thought to be the underlying cause. This explains the lower rate in those with gestational diabetes which classically occurs later than this, but not completely. Alterations in oxygen free radicals, myosinositol, and arachidonic acid metabolism and alterations in zinc metabolism have also been implicated.

The most common problem seen in the infant is macrosomia (in 8–50%), which can result in birth trauma and an increased intervention rate. As well as causing obesity, foetal hyperinsulinaemia also accelerates skeletal maturation, delays pulmonary maturation, and causes increased growth of insulin-sensitive tissues giving hypertrophy of the liver and heart. These infants also have an increased risk of hypoglycaemia, seen transiently in up to 50%, and jaundice, with rates of 6–50% quoted, and up to 50% of these requiring phototherapy. Polycythaemia is also seen.

Maternal

Maternal problems include an increased risk of infection and of pre-eclampsia, which is 2–3 times as likely to occur as in a non-diabetic mother.

Inheritance of diabetes

If the background rate of diabetes is 0.15%, the infant of a diabetic mother has a 2% rate and the infant of a diabetic father has a 6% rate. Interestingly the risk of type 2 diabetes in the child of a type 2 mother is much higher at 15–30%, rising to 50–60% if both parents have type 2 diabetes.

Known diabetics and pregnancy

Most women with diabetes have normal deliveries and normal babies. In most instances these are women with type 1 diabetes, although in some ethnic groups type 2 patients may make up a sizable group. In both groups it is sensible to have pre-conception glycaemic control optimized, e.g. preferably an HbAlc <7.0% or in the non-diabetic range. The congenital malformation and spontaneous abortion rates are significantly higher when the HbA1c is elevated. Once the HbA1c is 4–6 standard deviations above the normal non-diabetic range there is a fourfold increased in the malformation rate; at over 6 standard deviations above normal, this rises to a 12-fold risk. In the type 2 patients converting from oral agents to insulin is important. If not possible prior to conception it should be done as soon as a woman is found to be pregnant. Oral agents are potentially teratogenic and because of their ability to cross the placenta can further stimulate foetal β cells.

Pre-conception management

Pre-conception and post-conception advice is similar to that given to non-diabetic women, namely stopping smoking, reducing alcohol intake, avoiding unpasteurized dairy products, and adding oral folate supplements (5 mg/day). Reviewing the need for any.potentially teratogenic drugs they may be taking (e.g. antihypertensive agents usually), and what they can be swapped to, is also advised.

Ideally all patients who have diabetes and are pregnant should be managed in a combined clinic with an interested obstetrician. Reviews are initially 2–4 weekly then 1–2 weekly in the last third of pregnancy.

Maintain good glycaemic control

This is not just because of the risk of ketoacidosis which occurs in <l% of diabetic pregnancies and is associated with foetal loss in 20% of episodes, but also because of macrosomia in the foetus and both an increased foetal mortality (up to 2.2% of births in diabetic mothers) and an increased intervention rate at delivery. Aim to keep the glucose and HbAlc in the non-diabetic range to try to reduce the morbidity and mortality associated with pregnancy and diabetes. It should be remembered, however, that even with perfect control there is a small but significant excess of major congenital malformations in these children and an unexplained risk of late stillbirths.

Monitoring during pregnancy

* Capillary blood glucose monitoring is performed at least 4 times/day.

Target glycaemic control

* fasting glucoses of <5 mmol/L
* postprandial glucoses of <7 mmol/L
* keep the HbA1c in the non-diabetic range.

Treatment regimen

A basal bolus regimen gives greatest flexibility and is commonly used to achieve this target. In type 1 patients insulin requirements often fall in the first trimester, increase slightly in the second and then continue to rise until about 36 weeks, falling back to pre-pregnancy levels after delivery. In type 1 women remember early pregnancy is a cause of falling insulin requirements and recurrent hypoglycaemia. It has been suggested up to 40% of women with type 1 diabetes will experience significant hypoglycaemic episodes when pregnant and that hypoglycaemic awareness may alter. Advice regarding care with driving and other potentially hazardous pursuits is therefore needed early in pregnancy, if not before conception. Type 2 women requiring insulin usually need 0.9 units/kg per day initially and 1.6 units/kg per day later in the pregnancy.

Monitoring of diabetic complications during pregnancy

Certain diabetic complications are known to worsen during pregnancy, and screening for nephropathy and retinopathy in particular is advised at least each trimester.

Foetal monitoring

Scanning of the foetus is performed at 10–12 weeks looking for congenital abnormalities and to confirm dates. Repeat scanning to check for excessive growth/macrosomia at 18–20 weeks, 28 weeks, 32 weeks, and 36 weeks, although the exact timing and frequency can vary between centres.

Management of delivery

At delivery, most units have set protocols but, in general, induction soon after 38 weeks gestation (or not later than expected delivery date) and the use of a continuous insulin infusion with a separate dextrose and potassium infusion to maintain stable blood glucose levels is advisable. This is important as maternal hyperglycaemia during delivery can be associated with neonatal hypoglycaemia and an adverse neurological outcome in the infant.

After delivery

Monitoring of the infant with capillary blood glucoses post delivery is also often performed. The increased potential for hypoglycaemia in the mother and the baby if breast-feeding also needs watching out for, and extra carbohydrate snacks for the mother are often needed along with a 20–25% reduction in pre-conception insulin requirements. One day's worth of breast milk contains about 50 g of carbohydrate. Oral hypoglycaemic agents should not be recommended until after breast feeding has stopped.

Treatment regimen for labour/delivery

• If labour is induced, omit the previous evening's long acting insulin.

• Infuse 10% glucose at 75–125 mL/h (with 20 mmol potassium per 500 mL bag) .Infuse via a syringe driver 2–4 units/h of soluble insulin initially (usually made as 50 mL soluble insulin in 50 mL of 0.9% saline in a 50 mL syringe).

• Monitor capillary blood glucose levels hourly and adjust the infusion rate of the insulin to keep blood glucose levels in the 6–8 mmol/L range.

• Monitor fluid balance carefully (especially if oxytocin is also being given).

• Check serum sodium if labour lasts over 24 h (or 8 h with oxytocin)

After delivery

• Halve the i/v insulin infusion rate.

• Continue to monitor capillary blood glucose hourly for at least 4 h then 2–4 hourly until the mother is eating normally.

• Return to pre-pregnancy regimen when eating normally but be careful as insulin requirements can be low for the first 24 h.

Gestational diabetes

Epidemiology

Pregnancy potentially induces a state of insulin resistance with increases in the levels of growth hormone, progesterone, placental lactogen, and cortisol. This can therefore result in altered glucose handling. Impaired glucose tolerance during pregnancy occurs in up to 2–3% of pregnant women and may be associated with an increased risk of subsequent type 2 diabetes in 20–50% of patients. Worsening maternal insulin resistance and associated hyperglycaemia usually becomes evident from the second trimester onwards if it is going to occur.

As with women previously known to have diabetes, there is an association with worsening carbohydrate intolerance and a worse maternal and foetal outcome. Untreated gestational diabetes has been shown to have a perinatal mortality of 4.4–6.4% compared to 0.5–1.5% in a similar ethnic normoglycaemic population. Intensive insulin treatment has been shown to reduce such complications. This is the rationale for careful multidisciplinary care of these patients.

Treatment

Initial treatment is with dietary advice and in 10–30% insulin is also required. Insulin therapy should be considered if fasting blood glucoses are >6.0 mmol/L or post prandial levels are >8 mmol/L. Obesity is not uncommon and the importance of post-delivery dietary modification and weight reduction, to reduce the risk of future type 2 diabetes, should also be reinforced. The varying insulin requirements during pregnancy occur as in those with previously known diabetes, and most (but not all) will not need insulin treatment following delivery. Monitoring is with home capillary blood glucose measurements, daily if on diet alone and more frequently if on insulin therapy. The frequency needed depends on the results obtained with the aim to keep all readings <7.0 mmol/L. If diet alone fails, a basal bolus insulin regimen as used in the known diabetic is usually required. Decide on the total initial daily dose on the basis of the degree of hyperglycaemia present; 4–6 units per bolus is usual.

As with the previously known diabetic mother, the aim is to have a normal delivery , more often at 38 weeks to term depending on foetal growth. An oral glucose tolerance test 6 weeks after delivery is needed in all patients not requiring insulin post-delivery to confirm a return to normal glucose metabolism. A further reinforcement of diet and weight advice at this time is also usual practice. Whether these patients

Methods of screening

* Urine dip testing for glucose should be performed on every pregnant woman at every antenatal visit.
* If glycosuria is found a fasting glucose is performed and if >6.0 mmol/L a 75 g OGTT is needed.
* Routine screening at 28–32 weeks is also often performed, either with random blood glucoses or a fasting blood glucose and if a fasting level is >6.0 mmol/L or a postprandial level is >7.0 mmol/L an OGTT is required.
* The diagnostic criteria for diabetes are no different from those in the non-pregnant population. A diagnosis of gestational diabetes or gestational IGT is made if the fasting glucose is 6.0–7.8 mmol/L and/or the 2 h postprandial level is 9.0–11.0 mmol/L by the UK/St. Vincent definition. The WHO definition has a fasting level of 7.8 mmol/L and/or a 2 hour postprandial level of 7.8–11.1 mmol/L.

Table 8.1 Interpretation of the 75 g oral glucose tolerance test during pregnancy

	Plasma glucose (mmol/L)	
	Fasting	2 h proprandial level
Diabetes	>7.0	>11.0
Gestational IGT	6.0–7.8	9–11
Normal	<6.1	9

High risk groups

Most women are found on routine screening at about 30 weeks, but certain high risk groups should be screened earlier. These risk factors include:

* previous gestational diabetes
* a large baby in their last pregnancy, e.g. >4.0 kg at term
* a previous unexplained stillbirth/perinatal death
* maternal obesity
* family history of diabetes (first degree relatives)
* polyhydramnios.

should be followed up in view of their increased risk of diabetes is unclear at this time, but annual fasting blood glucose levels in asymptomatic women with a normal 6 week postpartum OGTT is often advised and more careful review is suggested in those with abnormal OGTTs.

Further reading

Dornhorst A, Chan SP. The elusive diagnosis of gestational diabetes. *Diabetic Medicine* 1998; 15: 7–10.

Garner P. Type 1 DM and pregnancy. *Lancet* 1995; 346: 157–161.

Girling JC, Dornhurst A. Pregnancy and diabetes mellitus. In Pickup J, Williams G (ed.) *Textbook of Diabetes,* 2nd edn, 72.1–34. Oxford: Blackwell Science, 1997.

Ilkova H. Screening for gestational diabetes. *Diabetes Reviews International* 1995; 3(3): 1–2.

Jardine Browne C *et al.* Pregnancy and neonatal care *Diabetic Medicine* 1996; 13: 843–853.

Contraception and diabetes

Oral contraceptives

The early combined oral contraceptive pills (OCP) impaired glucose tolerance and caused hyperinsulinism and so were not advised in patients with diabetes. The use of third-generation low-dose oestrogen-containing combined OCPs (e.g. 20 μg ethinyloestradiol) is safe in women <35 years of age. Third-generation OCPs are advised as they have a better risk profile for arterial disease and only occasionally increase insulin requirements.

As in the non-diabetic population, standard advice regarding the pill should be given and its avoidance in at-risk groups such as overweight smokers with a family history of thromboembolism and coronary heart disease is sensible. There is an increased risk of cerebral thromboembolism in type 1 patients, but the OCP dose not increase this.

In those with microvascular disease or coronary risk factors, the progesterone-only 'mini-pill' (POP) is safer than the combined OCP as it has no significant adverse effects on lipid metabolism, clotting, platelet aggregation, or fibrinolytic activity .It has been suggested that levonorgestrel- and norethisterone-containing POPs may reduce HDL2 cholesterol subfractions. The avoidance of POPs in those with established arterial disease is advised.

Barrier methods

The sheath and the diaphragm were historically the contraceptive method of choice in people with diabetes, and do not have the metabolic risks of the oral contraceptives described above. But, both are less effective forms of contraception with a failure rate of 0.7–3.6/00 couple years for the sheath and 2/100 couple years for the diaphragm, compared to nearly 0.2/100 women years with the combined OCP. In a population in which pregnancy carries significant risks, other forms of contraception are therefore now more often advocated.

Intrauterine contraceptive devices (IUD)

There is a concern that diabetes might make a pelvic infection associated with an IUD more severe and may render both copper containing and inert IUDs less effective, but not all studies have confirmed these worries. Nevertheless, if an IUD is used in a woman with diabetes a progestagen-releasing variety or a small copper device with regular use of spermicides are the current favourite options.

Hormone replacement therapy (HRT)

As with the OCP, diabetes itself is not a contraindication to the use of HRT. The oestrogens in HRT differ from those in the OCP and may actually reduce insulin resistance and also protect against coronary disease, although they may not actually reduce cardio-vascular events in those with established coronary artery disease.

Chapter 9
Intercurrent events or disease

Surgery

Preoperative assessment

Careful preoperative assessment is essential because of an increased risk of death and complications such as fluid overload from coronary heart disease and diabetic nephropathy. Any preoperative assessment in a patient with known diabetes should therefore include:

- an adequate history of diabetic complications
- a full examination looking for evidence of peripheral vascular disease, peripheral neuropathy, and lying/standing blood pressures in case of autonomic neuropathy
- assessment of current and overall diabetic control using blood glucose measurements in all patients and glycated haemoglobin.
- general investigations should include serum urea + electrolytes/ creatinine, full blood count, urine dip testing for protein, and an ECG (in anyone >45 years old).

Any further investigation will be based on problems found in the history or examination such as foot ulceration and potential osteomyelitis which may give a source for infection such as an MRSA.

Attempts should made to improve diabetic control, either on the ward or in a diabetic clinic, for any patient undergoing an elective procedure whose control is inadequate. An HbA1c <7.2% is considered good control, but an acceptable levels for most procedures would be <9%. Even with a good HbA1c level the preoperative glucose level (and if >11 mmol/L the urine ketones) should always be measured as the perioperative treatment is based on this and some stabilization before administration of an anaesthetic may be required, particularly in the emergency situation.

Perioperative management

Ideally patients with diabetes are best operated on in the morning at the start of the list.

Patients normally on diet alone should have their capillary blood glucose levels checked hourly and avoid i/v dextrose, and often need no other modification to their treatment. Patients taking oral agents should stop metformin preoperatively and miss their other agents on the morning of the procedure. If on chlorpropamide it should be missed the day before as well. Capillary blood glucose levels are again monitored regularly (1–2 hourly) and if >7.0 mmol/L start a dextrose + insulin regime as detailed below and aim to keep the glucose in the 7–11 mmol/L range.

Insulin regimens

Continuous i/v insulin infusion regimen/'sliding scale' insulin

50 units of soluble insulin in 50 mL 0.9% saline (giving 1 unit/mL) are placed in a 50 mL syringe and run through an automated syringe driver at a predetermined rate depending on regular capillary blood glucose measurements. Most units now have written guidelines for this type of regimen and each will need to be tailored to an individual patient, e.g. in insulin-resistant patients much larger amounts of insulin are needed. One such regimen is:

Blood glucose (mmol/L)	Insulin infusion rate (units/h or mL/h)
0–4.0	0.5 (+ recheck in 30 min)
4.1–7.0	1.0
7.1–11.0	2.0
11.1–17.0	4.0
>17.1	6.0–8.0 (+ review regimen)

I/v insulin regimens such as this should never be given without i/v fluids and potassium to avoid hypoglycaemia or hypokalaemia, e.g. start with 100 mL of 5% dextrose containing 5 mmol of potassium per hour. The postoperative rotating of dextrose and non-glucose containing i/v fluids can increase the risk of hypoglycaemia, especially if there is not careful monitoring of the blood glucose. Initially hourly capillary blood glucose levels are needed, moving to 2 hourly measurements postoperatively once stable results are obtained. An attempt at keeping the i/v dextrose infusion rate relatively constant makes this sort of regimen slightly safer. A preoperative potassium and daily repeat measurements are also required.

Postoperatively, once the patient has started eating adequately aim to revert back to a standard s/c insulin regimen with a premeal dose of insulin 30 min before food and the infusion stopping once this is working, i.e. when the food arrives. Patients previously on oral agents who require an i/v insulin regimen may have an increased insulin demand due to infection or the stress of the procedure and may require s/c insulin initially rather than just reverting to their preoperative oral agent(s), so be especially careful in this group.

The GIK regimen

Although not as popular as the above 'sliding scale' continuous regimen, this method does have the advantage of everything being given together so reducing the risk of insulin being given on its own. Into a 500 mL bag of 5% dextrose add 8 units of soluble

(cont.)

(*cont.*)

insulin and 5 mmol of potassium. Run this mixture at 100 mL/h and measure capillary blood glucoses hourly initially, aiming for levels of 7–11 mmol/L ideally and 5–15 mmol/L at worst. If >15 mmol/L, swap this infusion for one with 10 units of insulin but also check the serum potassium level to see if that also needs adjusting. If blood glucose is <5 mmol/L reduce the insulin to 6 units/500 mL of 5% dextrose. After each alteration recheck blood glucose levels after 1 h and adjust further if required. Once stable reduce the capillary blood glucose levels to 2 hourly. As with the other i/v regimen, convert to regular therapy once the patient is eating.

Certain situations may require further modification of this regimen, such as open heart surgery where the use of glucose-rich solutions and hypothermia can mean that higher doses of insulin are required initially.

In patients taking insulin undergoing a morning operation miss the morning insulin dose and start on a dextrose + insulin regimen as below. If on an afternoon list give half the normal morning dose of soluble insulin with a light breakfast and start the dextrose + insulin regimen at midday. Again aim to keep the blood glucose in the 7–11 mmol/L range.

Suitable insulin regimens

These come in two forms, the current favourite being a continuous i/v infusion adjusted on the basis of blood glucose measurements with a fixed dextrose infusion. The other is a single bag containing dextrose, insulin, and potassium known as the *Alberti regimen* or the *GIK (glucose insulin potassium) regimen* (opposite).

Skin/connective tissue/joint disease

Skin

Diabetes results in an increased occurrence of infections such as vaginal candida, candida balanitis, and *Staphylococcus aureus* folliculitis. Ulceration in the feet due to neuropathy and peripheral vascular disease should also be considered. Other skin features to look for include the following.

Conditions specific to diabetes

- pretibial diabetic dermopathy ('shin spots')
- diabetic bullae (bullosis diabeticorum, very rare tense blistering on feet/lower legs classically)
- diabetic thick skin (scleroderma of diabetes seen in 2.5% with type 2 diabetes)
- periungual telangectasia (venous capillary dilatation at the nail fold seen in up to 50% of people with diabetes).

Conditions seen more commonly in those with diabetes

- necrobiosis lipoidica
- vitiligo (seen in 2% with type 1 diabetes)
- granuloma annulare (though this association is not proven conclusively).

Conditions associated with the other biochemical features seen in diabetes

- acanthosis nigricans (with insulin resistance)
- eruptive xanthomata (with hypertriglyceridaemia).

The most common skin lesion in diabetes are shin spots or diabetic dermopathy. These occur more commonly in men than in women and affect up to 50% of people with diabetes. Their aetiology is uncertain. They present initially as red papules and progress to give well circumscribed atrophic areas, brownish in colour. Usually seen on the shins, they can also be found on the forearms and thighs. There is no effective treatment of these but they usually resolve spontaneously over 1–2 years.

Necrobiosis lipoidica is seen in 0.3–1% of people with diabetes, and 40–60% of those with necrobiosis also have diabetes. It is more common in women than in men. Classically seen on the shins, it has an atrophic centre with telangectasia around the edge of an oval or irregular lesion, although early lesions can be dull red plaques or papules. Treatment with topical or injectable steroids may help improve these lesions; skin grafting and cosmetic camouflage have also been used.

When looking at the skin do not forget to check injection sites for lipohypertrophy or lipoatrophy as these are often much more amenable to treatment or correction. In the past an insulin allergy rash was also commonly seen, but more recently a transient local reaction, thought to be an IgE-mediated reaction, is more often seen.

Connective tissue/joint disease

Diabetes is associated with an increased incidence of pseudogout and osteoarthritis, but the classical condition to consider is the 'stiff hand syndrome' or *diabetic cheiroarthropathy*. In this the skin thickens and tightens which, in association with sclerosis of the tendon sheaths, results in limited joint mobility in the hands and less commonly the feet. This reduced joint mobility gives an inability to place the palms of the hand flat together and make the 'prayer sign'. No specific treatment for this currently exists.

Chapter 10

Social and practical aspects

Current regulations for fitness to drive motor vehicles

Diabetes is said to influence the ability to drive safely because of hypo-glycaemia or complications such as a reduction in vision acuity or fields. It carries a similar risk of accidents to epilepsy (e.g. relative risk of 1.23–1.24 compared to standard drivers). The Driver and Vehicle Licensing Agency (DVLA) Drivers Medical Unit produced a revised set of guidelines in February 1999, which are outlined below.

A group 1 licence is the standard motorcycle/motor car licence (e.g. categories A and B) which also allows you to drive a private minibus carrying up to 16 people (category D1) or a vehicle between 3.5 and 7.5 tonnes (category C1). A group 2 licence allows you to drive heavy goods vehicles (HGVs) and passenger carrying vehicles (PCVs), and all holders of these must inform the DVLA of their diabetes what ever their treatment.:

- Any patient with uncomplicated diabetes who is on *diet alone* does not need to inform the DVLA unless they live in Northern Ireland, they develop complications which will interfere with their ability to drive, or their therapy changes.

- Women who develop *gestational diabetes* need to inform the DVLA and must re-inform them 6 weeks after delivery if still on insulin. They must also stop driving while pregnant if their control is poor and automatically lose their group 2 licence until after delivery.

- *Insulin-treated patients* are required to inform the DVLA if they are on insulin therapy and will need to renew their licences every 1–3 years. They must demonstrate satisfactory control, recognize warning symptoms of hypoglycaemia, and have acceptable eyesight for a standard group 1 licence. New applicants for a driving licence or existing drivers starting on insulin do not automatically get a C1 + D1 licence. From 11/9/98 some previous licence holders, subject to annual review, can keep their class C1 vehicle licence for 3.5–7.5 tonne lorries, but not for D1. Since 1991 they were also barred from driving HGVs or PCVs. Drivers licensed before 1/4/91 who are on insulin are reassessed annually and may still do so.

- *Patients managed with tablets* need to inform the DVLA and can normally continue to hold both a group 1 (until 70 years old) and a group 2 licence, subject to a satisfactory medical. If vision deterio-rates, hypoglycaemia is a problem, or they require insulin therapy this may alter.

Travel

Travel across time zones, exposure to unaccustomed exercise, and new infections make this an important area for both patient and doctor education. It is common sense to take more insulin than is needed for any time away, in case of an accidental loss or breakage. If new insulin supplies are needed, remember not all countries use only the U100 strength and tell the patient travelling abroad to look out for this, e.g 30 units or 0.3 mL of U100 strength insulin equates to 0.75 mL of the U40 form and 0.38 mL of U80. A letter stating the need to carry insulin, needles, and syringes/pen devices will also make Customs formalities slightly easier.

Patients with diabetes need the same immunizations and malaria prophylaxis as other travellers. In case they acquire an infection or illness while travelling, standard 'sick day rules' should be reinforced. These suggest that:

• Insulin therapy should never be stopped and may actually need to be increased, even when food intake is reduced.

• If the patient is unable to tolerate solid food, a liquid form of carbohydrate such as Lucozade or Dioralyte should be taken instead. A patient who is unable to tolerate adequate oral fluids should seek medical advice.

• If unwell monitor urine for ketones and if present seek medical advice.

• During any illness consider increasing the frequency of capillary glucose testing.

Travel and adjustments in therapy are usually more of a problem for insulin-treated patients as those on oral agents can adjust the timing of their tablets to the new time zone with less risk of significant deteriorations in control.

In the insulin-treated patient:

• On short flights where the differences in time zones is small no major insulin adjustments are needed, but make sure snacks and extra carbohydrate are packed with hand luggage as the timing, quality, and quantity of airline food is rather variable.

• On longer flights where time zones are crossed the adjustments needed will depend on their initial regimen and the direction of travel. If travelling east to west the day is longer and extra doses are needed; west to east gives a shorter day and so a reduction in therapy is required. With a basal bolus regimen take soluble insulin with each meal given and intermediate acting insulin given to fit in with the evening at the destination. In a twice daily mixed regimen give an extra dose of soluble when going east to west and miss the evening isophane when going west to east.

(cont.)

(*cont.*)

Exercise

Non-diabetic people initially breakdown muscle glycogen for 5–10 min, then use circulating glucose and non-esterified fatty acids. Hepatic glucose production increases, but free fatty acids are the main fuel used after 1–2 h of exercise and without some form of energy intake most people become hypoglycaemic after 2–3 h of strenuous exercise. Insulin sensitivity also decreases the day after severe exertion.

Type 1 diabetes

Insulin requirements are reduced during exercise. To reduce the risk of hypoglycaemia with acute exercise decrease the pre-exercise insulin dose, which would have its peak during the exercise, by 30–50%. If the exercise is due to last more than 2 h also take 20–40 g of extra carbohydrate before and hourly during exercise.

If the site of the insulin injection is the area being exercised absorption may be accelerated, especially if exercise is undertaken soon after the injection of an insulin analogue. So inject into an area that won't be exercised. With extreme exercise it may take several hours, if not until the next day, to fully replenish muscle glycogen stores and care is needed to avoid hypoglycaemia during this period.

Type 2 diabetes

Exercise increases peripheral glucose uptake and reduces endogenous insulin secretion. Physical training can increase insulin sensitivity which in type 2 patients can result in a reduction in HbA1c, blood pressure, weight, and a better lipid profile. Hypoglycaemia is not usually a problem unless the patient is taking sulfonylureas, so extra carbohydrate is not normally indicated. In those using these agents a reduction in dosage may however be advisable.

Complications from diabetes and driving

Loss of hypoglycaemic awareness will result in permanent loss of an HGV/PCV licence and a temporary loss of a standard licence until specialist reports can confirm that awareness has returned. Any doctor making this diagnosis must tell the patient they are legally obliged to inform the DVLA of this diagnosis. If the patient refuses to do so the medical adviser at the DVLA should be informed once the patient has been informed in writing of the intention to do so. Avoiding all hypoglycaemic episodes for at least a month will help to regain hypoglycaemic awareness in some patients. A patient who is unable to regain this awareness *must* stop driving.

In a patient with frequent hypoglycaemic episodes or with poor control it seems sensible to advise them not to drive until things are better, and the DVLA should be contacted. As part of their regular checks the DVLA asks a doctor to complete a Diabetes III form which asks if control of the diabetes is satisfactory/stable and how long this has been for. This should help to pick up many of these patients. If you say their control is poor or unstable, do not forget to tell the patient what you have done and arrange to see them to improve this problem as reports to that effect will be needed by the DVLA before their licence is renewed.

Visual requirements are that you can read a number plate with 79.4 mm high letters at 20.5 m with glasses/contact lenses if worn. This equates to a visual acuity of between 6/9 and 6/12 on a Snellen chart. Group 2 licence holders must have an acuity of 6/9 or better in their good eye and not worse than 6/12 in the bad, but will not be licenced if they have an uncorrected acuity worse than 3/60 in either eye. Visual field defects of any sort, especially if bilateral, result in loss of HGV/PCV licences and may affect a standard licence.

Other complications such as limb amputations can alter the ability to drive, but driving is still possible if the vehicle is suitably modified.

Useful addresses

DVLA (Driver and Vehicle Licensing Agency), Drivers Medical Unit, Longview
Road, Morriston, Swansea SA99 1DA. Tel: 01792 783795. Fax: 01792 783687
Diabetes U.K, 10 Queen Anne Street, London W1M 0BD.
Tel 020 7323 1531. BDA motor insurance quote line: 01903 262 900

Chapter 11
Emergencies in diabetes

Diabetic ketoacidosis

Diabetic ketoacidosis has a mortality of 2–5%. Many deaths occur due to delays in presentation and initiation of treatment, with a mortality rate of up to 50% in the elderly.

Diagnosis

This is usually based on a collection of biochemical abnormalities, namely:

- *hyperglycaemia* >11.1 mmol/L
- *acidosis* arterial pH <7.3, serum bicarbonate <15 mmol/L, base excess <−10
- *ketonuria* Some dip testing methods only check for acetoacetate and acetone but not β-hydroxybutyrate. Captopril can also give a false positive test for urinary acetone. Ketones may also interfere with some creatinine assays and give falsely high readings.

There is an uncommon condition of *euglycaemic ketoacidosis* (in 1–3% of cases at most) when ketones are produced early on in patients with a reduced carbohydrate intake. Blood glucose is <17 mmol/L, acidosis is marked, and dehydration is not usually severe. Treatment is to initiate oral carbohydrate intake and monitor the need for i/v insulin/fluids as in full-blown hyperglycaemic ketoacidosis.

Epidemiology

Diabetic ketoacidosis is common in type 1 patients, with 1 in 11 subjects in the European IDDM complications study (EURODIAB) reporting hospitalization for this over a 12 month period. The incidence is 5–8/1000 diabetic patients per year, usually type 1 patients but up to 25% of cases are patients with newly diagnosed/presenting diabetes some of whom subsequently obtain adequate control with oral agents or diet alone. In up to 50% of cases an infection is the precipitant and in 10–30% of cases it is their first presentation with diabetes.

Pathogenesis

Diabetic ketoacidosis occurs as a result of insulin deficiency and counterregulatory hormone excess. Insulin deficiency results in excess mobilization of free fatty acids from adipose tissue. This provides the substrate for ketone production from the liver. Ketones (β-hydroxybutyrate, acetoacetate, and acetone) are excreted by the kidneys and buffered in the blood initially, but once this system fails acidosis develops. Hyperglycaemia also occurs as the liver produces glucose from

Precipitants of diabetic ketoacidosis

infection	30–40%
non-compliance with treatment	25%
inappropriate alterations in insulin (i.e. errors by patient or doctor)	13%
newly diagnosed diabetes	10–20%
myocardial infarction	1%

lactate and alanine which are generated by muscle proteinolysis. The reduced peripheral glucose utilization associated with insulin deficiency exacerbates this.

Hyperglycaemia and ketonuria cause an osmotic diuresis and hypovolaemia with both intracellular and extracellular dehydration. Glomerular filtration is reduced and blood glucose levels therefore rise even further as do the levels of counterregulatory hormones such as glucagon. The metabolic acidosis due to ketone accumulation leads to widespread cell death which combined with hypovolaemia is fatal if untreated.

Clinical features

Polyuria, polydypsia, and weight loss are often seen. Muscle cramps, abdominal pain, and shortness of breath (air hunger or Kussmaul's breathing, with deep regular rapid breaths, suggesting acidosis) can also occur. Subsequent nausea and vomiting can worsen both the dehydration and electrolyte losses which often precede the onset of coma (occuring in about 10% of cases). Remember to consider other causes of coma and a raised blood glucose such as head injury, alcohol, and drug overdoses.

On examination the breath can smell of ketones (like nail varnish remover) with postural hypotension (exacerbated by peripheral vasodilatation due to acidosis) and hypothermia also frequently seen. Infection and trauma can precipitate this problem and should be carefully looked for, especially in the unconscious patient.

Hypovolaemia at presentation is usually at least 5 L with electrolyte losses of 300–700 mmol of sodium, 200–700 mmol of potassium, and 350–500 mmol of chloride accompanying this. The daily intake of both sodium and potassium is 60 mmol, so the severity of this is apparent.

Management

Having first assessed the need for immediate resuscitation, and commenced a 0.9% saline i/v infusion, take a history and examine the patient to look for obvious precipitants such as surgery, trauma, sites of infection, or myocardial infarction. Initial investigations will be modified by the history and examination and suggested site of infection but should at least include:

- blood for urea/electrolytes (note ketone/creatinine assay interaction)
- full blood count (a leukocytosis can occur without infection)
- arterial blood gases (P_aCO_2 will be low due to hyperventilation with a metabolic acidosis, check pH and bicarbonate)
- cultures of blood and urine
- chest radiograph and ECG

Initial treatment of ketoacidosis

I/v 0.9% saline

- 2 L in 2 h then 1 L over 2 h, 2 L in next 8 h and 4 L/day thereafter until blood glucose <11 mmol/L. Then convert to dextrose saline or 5% dextrose.
- If the patient is profoundly shocked (e.g. systolic BP <80 mmHg with severe dehydration or sepsis) or oliguric, this may need to be given more rapidly and colloids may also be needed. If elderly or there are signs of heart failure or cerebral oedema this may need to be given more slowly.

Potassium

Once the serum potassium is known the 0.9% saline has potassium added with the dose adjusted based on hourly serum potassium measurements until stable and measured 2–4 hourly over the next 12–24 h. Add:

- 40 mmol/L if K$^+$ <3.0 mmol/L
- 30 mmol/L if K$^+$ 3.0–4.0 mmol/L
- 20 mmol/L if K$^+$ 4.1–5.0 mmol/L
- 10 mmol/L if K$^+$ 5.1–6.0 mmol/L
- none if K$^+$ >6.0 mmol/L.

Insulin (via a continuous i/v infusion)

- 50 units of soluble insulin in 50 mL of 0.9% saline given at 6–8 units/hour to drop glucose by about 5 mmol/L per hour and adjusted to keep blood glucose 10–14 mmol/L until after ketoacidosis has cleared (usually need 3–6 units/hour).
- Alternatively use 50 units of insulin in 500 mL of 0.9% saline with added potassium infused at 80–100 mL/hour initially with a maintenance dose of 30–60 mL/hour once blood glucose is adequately controlled. I/m regimes should be avoided and used only as a last resort. Give 20 units of soluble insulin initially with 10 units hourly until blood glucose falls and then 20 units 6 hourly until control is achieved.

- in the older patient (>40 years) also include an ECG and cardiac enzymes, even if asymptomatic.

Replacement of fluids, electrolytes, and insulin is the mainstay of treatment, along with treating any precipitant, such as infection. To monitor this treatment central venous access and urinary catheterization are often necessary and a nasogastric tube may be useful, especially in the unconscious patient. In elderly people, those with a cardiac history, or those with autonomic neuropathy central venous access is imperative.

Monitoring

Once treatment has commenced, monitor fluid balance carefully and avoid fluid overload. Check capillary blood glucose hourly with serum potassium, sodium, and glucose 2 hourly and arterial blood gases 2–4 hourly depending on response. Reduce the frequency of tests once stabilized but check electrolytes at least daily for the first 72 h. Continuous ECG monitoring will aid the detection of hypo- and hyperkalaemia in the acute phase. Magnesium and phosphate levels should also be checked as these can occasionally require replacement therapy.

Additional therapies

- *I/v bicarbonate* is only rarely indicated as it can cause hypokalaemia and paradoxically worsen intracellular acidosis. If used, give only when the pH is <6.9 using 250 mL of 1.26% bicarbonate given over 30–60 min initially and monitor arterial blood gases to assess response, aiming for pH no greater than 7.1. This should probably only be used in an intensive care setting. Do not use 8.4% bicarbonate as its high sodium load can too rapidly alter electrolyte levels and precipitate pulmonary oedema as well as causing local tissue necrosis if it extravasates.

- In severe hypotension unresponsive to colloids and crystalloids inotropes may be required but agents such as *dopamine*, *dobutamine*, and *adrenaline* will all exacerbate insulin resistance necessitating a more aggressive sliding scale regime.

- *Heparin* in s/c prophylactic doses can be given in the unconscious or immobile patent.

- Cover with *i/v broad-spectrum antibiotics* should be used if no obvious precipitant is found and appropriate antibiotics if a site of infection is found.

- Cerebral oedema typically presents 8–24 h after starting i/v fluids with a declining conscious level and may have a mortality as high as 90%. If this occurs *dexamethasone* (12–16 mg/day) and *mannitol* (1–2 g/kg body weight) may be given.

Subsequent treatment

Once the blood glucose is stable in the 10–15 mmol/L range, the ketoacidosis has settled, and the patient is eating and drinking normally consider swapping on to a s/c insulin regime but overlap the i/v and the first s/c dose by 2 h. Stabilize on this therapy before discharge from hospital. Once the i/v potassium supplements have stopped, give oral supplements for at least 48 h with regular serum monitoring.

Patient education to determine the cause and so avoid a further occurrence, or for earlier presentation if it does occur, should also ideally be performed before discharge.

Hyperosmolar, non-ketotic hyperglycaemia

This is a more sinister complication than ketoacidosis with a mortality as high as 50% and is said to be found in 11–30% of adult hyperglycaemic emergencies. It affects an older population than ketoacidosis (middle aged or elderly), 2/3 of cases are in patients with previously undiagnosed diabetes, and its insidious onset can be mistaken for many other conditions including a stroke.

Diagnosis

This is again a biochemical diagnosis:

- *hyperglycaemia* (usually 30–70 mmol/L)
- serum osmolality *high* (> 350 mmol/kg)
- *no acidosis* arterial pH 7.35–7.45, serum bicarbonate >18 mmol/L, but remember lactic acidosis with infection or a myocardial infarction may alter this.
- *no ketonuria* + on urine dip testing can occur with starvation and vomiting.

Serum osmolality (in mosmol/kg) can be calculated if not available from the laboratory using the following equation:

osmolality = 2(sodium + potassium) + glucose + urea

Epidemiology

This occurs in an older age group of insulin-producing type 2 patients, a large proportion of whom will not previously be known to have diabetes. Ingestion of high-sugar-containing drinks, intercurrent infection, and myocardial infarction are all commonly seen as precipitants of this condition. Drugs such as glucocorticoids, cimetidine, phenytion, thiazide, and loop diuretics have all been implicated in the pathogenesis of this problem.

Pathogenesis

This occurs from a combination of insulin deficiency and counter-regulatory hormone excess with the insulin present stopping ketone production but in insufficient quantities to prevent worsening hyperglycaemia.

Clinical features

There is normally an insidious onset with several days of ill-health and profound dehydration at presentation (equivalent to a 9–10 L deficit).

Confusion is not uncommon, nor is coma (especially once serum osmolality >440) and occasionally fits occur. Gastroparesis and associated vomiting with gastric erosions and subsequent haematemesis can occur. These patients are also hypercoagulable, and venous thromboses and cerebrovascular events are important to exclude.

Management

Initial investigation and treatment is the same as for ketoacidosis with fluid, electrolyte and insulin replacement, although there are a few important exceptions as these are older patients:

- The fluid regime should be less rapid/vigorous. Central venous access for monitoring is more often required. e.g. 1 L of 0.9% saline over the first hour, 1 L 2 hourly for the next 2 h, then 1 L 4–6 hourly.

- If hypernatraemic (serum sodium >155 mmol/L) consider 0.45% saline, rather than 0.9% although this may increase the risk of cerebral oedema if serum sodium or osmolality is altered too rapidly as it has a mortality as high as 70%.

- Prophylactic s/c heparin should be considered, although recent evidence suggests more formal anticoagulation carries a high risk of upper gastrointestinal bleeding.

- A gentler insulin regime is needed with 3–6 units/h of soluble insulin i/v aiming to reduce the blood glucose by a maximum of 5 mmol/h to avoid precipitating cerebral oedema.

- A more aggressive use of i/v antibiotics is encouraged.

Subsequent treatment

Continue i/v fluids and insulin for at least 24 h after initial stabilization and then convert to maintenance therapy such as s/c insulin or oral hypoglycaemic agents. Patient education to avoid further episodes is also advisable.

Hypoglycaemia

This complication of the treatment of diabetes should be excluded in any unconscious or fitting patient. If prolonged it can result in death. Most insulin-treated patients can expect to experience hypoglycaemic episodes at some time, with up to 1/7 having a more severe episode each year and 3% suffering recurrent episodes. The 25% of people on long term insulin who lose their hypoglycaemic awareness are of particular concern. Nocturnal hypoglycaemic episodes with a hyperglycaemic response the next morning (due to increased counter-regulatory hormones – the Somogyi phenomenon), which tend to occur in younger insulin-treated patients, should not be forgotten and may only present with morning headaches or a drunken feeling.

Diagnosis

This is a biochemical diagnosis from a blood glucose <2.5 mmol/L but is often first picked up by the patient, their family, or their doctor from the clinical features below. Saving serum before treatment for blood glucose, insulin, and C-peptide levels will confirm the diagnosis and may help determine the cause.

Pathogenesis

Hypoglycaemia results from an imbalance between glucose supply, glucose utilization, and insulin levels resulting in more insulin than is needed at that time. A reduced glucose supply occurs when a meal or snack is missed, or as a late effect of alcohol. It can also be due to delayed gastric emptying with autonomic neuropathy or be associated with coeliac disease, Addison's disease, or an acute illness, such as gastroenteritis. Increased utilization occurs with exercise and high insulin levels mostly with sulfonylurea or exogenous insulin therapy. The net result of this imbalance is hypoglycaemia.

Human insulins have a slightly faster onset of action and a shorter duration of action than their animal predecessors, and a lot of patients report alterations in hypoglycaemic awareness when they switch from one to the other. Even so, no definite evidence of specific hypoglycaemic alterations due to human insulin itself have been reported.

Sulfonylurea therapy can cause hypoglycaemia due to β cell stimulation. This is most commonly seen from *glibenclamide*, especially in the elderly and those with reduced renal excreting ability, but can occur in anyone who takes this therapy and fasts, especially with longer acting agents such as *chlorpropamide*.

The biguanide *metformin* and the α-glucosidase inhibitor *acarbose* are unlikely to precipitate hypoglycaemia, but insulin-sensitizing

Signs and symptoms of hypoglycaemia

Autonomic

* sweating
* pallor
* anxiety
* nausea
* tremor
* shivering
* palpitations
* tachycardia

Neuroglycopaenia

* confusion
* tiredness
* lack of concentration
* headache
* dizziness
* altered speech
* incoordination
* drowsiness
* aggression
* coma

agents such as the ACEIs and newer agents such as the thiazolidine-diones (e.g. *rosiglitazone*) may do so.

Clinical features

The features of hypoglycaemia can be divided into two main groups: autonomic symptoms and neuroglycopenic symptoms, as shown on p. 119. The autonomic symptoms usually occur first (when the blood glucose <3.6 mmol/L), but some drugs such as the non-selective β-blockers and alcohol may mask these with neuroglycopenia (at blood glucose <2.6 mmol/L) then causing confusion with no warning. Some patients lose these predominantly autonomic warning symptoms and are therefore at higher risk of injury.

Management

In the conscious patient, oral carbohydrate (20–30 g) is often sufficient to resolve the problem. This can be given as 5–6 dextrosol tablets or as a glass of milk or orange juice. Having raised the sugar rapidly then give something to maintain a normal blood glucose level such as two digestive biscuits. In the confused patient a buccal gel (e.g. hypostop, a 30% glucose gel) is an alternative although this should not be used in the unconscious patient as there is a risk of aspiration.

In the unconscious patient, once a blood sample has been taken for glucose estimation, treat with 25–50 mL of 50% dextrose i/v or 1 mg of i/m or deep s/c glucagon. Glucagon mobilizes glycogen from the liver and will not work if given repeatedly or in starved patients with no glycogen stores. In this situation or if prolonged treatment is needed, i/v glucose is better (50% initially then 10%).

Subsequent management

Having corrected the acute event determine why it happened and, if possible, alter treatment or lifestyle to stop it recurring. Extreme exercise may require an alteration in insulin doses for 24 h, and alcohol causes not only initial hyperglycaemia but also a degree of hypo-glycaemia 3–6 h after ingestion, and may alter insulin requirements the next morning. Education to avoid precipitating hypoglycaemic episodes in these situations is advisable. Recurrent hypoglycaemic events may also herald a deterioration in renal or liver function and these should be excluded.

Further reading

Amiel SA, Tamborlane WV, Sherwin RS. Defective glucose counterregulation after strict glycaemic control of insulin-dependent DM. *New England Journal of Medicine* 1987; 316: 1376–1384.

Cranston ICP, Amiel SA. Hypoglycaemia. In: Leslie RDG, Robbins DC, ed. *Diabetes: Clinical Science and Practice.* Cambridge: Cambridge University Press, 1995: 375–391.

Frier B. Hypoglycaemia in DM. In Pickup J, Williams G, ed. *Textbook of Diabetes*, 2nd edn. Oxford: Blackwell Science, 1997.

Hepburn D, Deary IJ, Frier BM *et al.* Symptoms of acute insulin induced hypoglycaemia in humans with and without IDDM. *Diabetes Care* 1991; 14: 949–957.

Krentz AJ, Nattrass M. Acute metabolic complications of DM: diabetic ketoacidosis, hyperosmolar non-ketotic syndrome and lactic acidosis. In Pickup J, Williams G, ed. *Textbook of Diabetes*, 2nd edn. Oxford: Blackwell Science, 1997: 39.1–23.

Lebovitz HE. Diabetic ketoacidosis. *Lancet* 1995; 345: 767–772.

Appendix:
Patient support groups

Useful addresses (UK)

Diabetes UK
10 Queen Anne Street, London, W1M 0BD

Useful addresses overseas

American Diabetes Association
1701 North Beauregard Street,
Alexandria, VA 22311, USA

Useful web sites

www.diabetes.org.uk   Diabetes UK

www.diabetes.org   American Diabetes Association

Index